REVIEWS

As both a polio survivor and a retired occupational therapist, I am well aware of the state of the American Medical System. I've watched it deteriorate, more than improve, over the last few decades. With our high level of technology and research, this is unacceptable! It's high time our people are educated on this reality. I have long been enraged seeing our medical system putting a bandaid over a festering wound to cover it up, then pretending that's enough…without actually resolving/healing/seeking/treating the actual core and cause of the disease. We must be willing to look deeper, multilevel-mind, body, emotions, soul -then care enough to resolve and prevent the root cause of the disease in our society! We do, indeed, live in a "sickness" society rather than a wellness society. Healthcare for profit is NOT working, nor sustainable for our medical system, and definitely NOT serving the people! I've recently seen both nurses and CNA's in a state of overwhelm, experiencing burn-out, unable to continue working, or even quitting their jobs and choosing a different career for their own survival, just when they are needed most. It is a sad thing to watch or experience this under-staffing when you are the one needing the help. Well done, Traci-our world is ready for transparency and for the truth to be revealed!! Your book is full of good suggestions and resources to empower and enable people to self-advocate for better medical communications and results.

Laurel Tinney, OT retired

A great read, and very important information that everyone should be aware of. Being a nurse in this system as well, she nails the most important aspects of what you should know. Definitely worth the time to read, it may save your life one day.

Cyndi Hall, RN

SURVIVE THE HOSPITAL

BE YOUR OWN ADVOCATE

TRACI KONAS & TAMMY BERGSTROM

Survive The Hospital • Be Your Own Advocate • Don't Get Neglected

Copyright © 2023 Traci Konas

ISBN 9798218125899

DEDICATION

*Dedicated to my father, who died due to negligence
at Northridge Hospital on 08/26/17 @ 0017
hours and to my mother who lost half her nose
because the doctor wouldn't listen to her.*

Have you ever walked out of the doctor's office wondering what just happened?

Have you left the hospital in worse condition than before you went in?

Have you lost a family member or a friend knowing the hospital made a mistake or felt like they did make a mistake?

Have you been denied a medical procedure or treatment because your insurance company refused to pay for it?

Are you frustrated by the system, feeling ignored, inundated with medical bills, or completely lost when you go see a doctor?

Well, you're not alone! My name is Traci, I have been an emergency room Nurse for 12 years, along with many other specialties. I lost my father due to the negligence of our system and my mother lost half her nose because the doctor wouldn't listen to her, which is why I'm writing this book.

I will teach you about how our healthcare system works, offer some solutions to help change it, and show you how to be your own advocate. I'm going to tell you what really goes on, on the inside!

I am going to give you pointers on how to survive while in the hospital, maintain a healthier lifestyle so you don't end up in the hospital, how to interact with your doctor, what test results mean, and how to demand care and actually get it.

I had a doctor recently tell me, "Do you want to survive? Don't go to the hospital." We all know we will end up there one day. So be prepared when you do!

Empower yourself with knowledge!

CONTENTS

PART

1

A Death That Never Needed To Happen

On August 26, 2017, I received a text that no son or daughter wants to receive.

"Your dad is in the Intensive Care Unit (ICU). You need to get here as soon as you can," my stepmother said with heaviness in her voice.

"The ICU?! I didn't even know he was in the hospital! Why didn't you tell me?!" I said, appalled by how I'd been left out of the loop during this critical time.

I drove as fast as I could to Northridge Hospital and tried my best to prepare myself for what I was about to see. I didn't know what to expect, but I knew it was going to be bad and I had a terrible feeling.

My father had been in and out of the hospital for about

a month due to his emphysema and more recently for pneumonia. He was only 62 and didn't have a laundry list of issues. He was a smoker, hence the emphysema, but nothing serious beyond that.

He had been complaining of having trouble breathing for at least a month leading up to this and medical staff didn't seem to be too concerned. He received antibiotics for his pneumonia, but they didn't work. He had to come back into the emergency room yet again because he could not catch his breath.

In the emergency room I worked in, when we admitted someone with pneumonia who had an elevated heart rate, blood pressure, and potassium levels, along with reduced kidney function like my dad did, we would send them to the telemetry unit at the minimum.

Elevated levels of potassium in the blood can indicate kidney failure, can cause a heart attack, and should be taken seriously. Because pneumonia is notorious for turning deadly fast, a telemetry unit is the base level of care for these patients.

A telemetry unit is where patients go who need constant monitoring. The patient's vitals are taken every 4 hours, they are always hooked up to a heart monitor, and the patient-to-nurse ratio is 4 to 1 (in California) for better monitoring if anything changes. This is where my dad should have been, but he was not.

Instead, he was sent to the medical/surgical unit where patients get much less monitoring. This unit is meant to be somewhat of a holding area for palliative care and people recovering from basic surgery. In fact, vitals are only taken every 12 hours and the patient's heart is not continuously monitored. When a patient is having trouble breathing, is suffering from pneumonia, and is having signs of kidney failure, they should be closely watched... but my dad was not.

He continued to degrade throughout the day, was put on a Bi-pap machine to help him breathe, yet still wasn't transferred to the telemetry unit! The last set of vitals were taken that night at 9pm, which showed tachycardia (fast heart rate) and *not again until the next morning at 6am! No one even checked on him until the next morning!*

When they checked him that next morning, he was barely breathing. In fact, he was barely alive. A rapid response team was called who intubated him and took him to the ICU. They hooked him up to a ventilator to help him breathe, inserted a PICC (peripherally inserted central catheter) line for IV fluids, and started to administer blood pressure medications to prevent his blood pressure from dropping too low.

By the time I arrived at the hospital and rushed into the ICU, I took one look at my dad and knew he was not going to make it. With so much experience dealing with death in the ER, I had gotten rather good at looking at someone and knowing about how long they had to live. When I looked at my dad, I knew he would die that night. *I had gotten there too late.*

He was mottled (turning purple), his blood pressure was terribly low (even though he was on 3 blood pressure medications), he was tachycardic at 150 BPM (high heart rate), oxygenation of his blood was 88%, and all his labs indicated that he was severely septic. Sepsis is a life-threatening condition where your body is trying to fight an infection that has spread to your bloodstream. As sepsis worsens, blood flow to the vital organs such as the heart, brain, and kidneys are impaired, and they start to die.

"Why haven't you put an arterial line in yet?" I asked his doctor angrily.

"He doesn't need one yet," was the doctor's reply.

"Doesn't need one? He's purple! How much worse does he have to get?!" I exclaimed. I couldn't believe these doctors were so nonchalant about my father's life. The doctor, of course, hurried away as if he had something important to do and never acted on my question.

An arterial line has more functionality than a PICC line. A PICC line administers fluids and medication through a flexible catheter in your arm, which gets threaded close to the heart. An arterial line allows for much more detailed information regarding blood pressure, acid/base balance, and body temperature. He also lacked a central line; It has 3 ports to administer 3 different medications at one time and given its location close to the heart, medication enters the bloodstream within seconds and the heart pumps it to the rest of the body.

All these devices are essential when dealing with a critical care patient like my dad.

On top of that, one of the three blood pressure medications they had him on causes tachycardia and his heart rate was 150-170 BPM for hours. That's when I asked heatedly, "Why don't we put him on another blood pressure medication that *doesn't* cause tachycardia *before* you *give* him a *heart attack*, and why haven't you started him on dialysis yet?! He has kidney failure now and the high potassium will give him a heart attack! Don't you have ECMO?!" I requested that he be transferred via helicopter to a hospital that did have ECMO (extracorporeal membrane oxygenation) and competent staff but they said he probably wouldn't survive the flight and my stepmother wouldn't agree with the transfer.

So why didn't his doctor put an arterial and central line in him upon being admitted to the ICU that morning? Obviously, he was in critical condition, yet not even the bare minimum was being done. At my hospital, it was one of the first things we did with a severely septic patient.

After getting no help from the doctor I talked to when I first arrived, another doctor started their shift and took over the care of my dad. She had some reasoning abilities and was receptive to putting an arterial and a central line in, along with adjusting the medications and adding a catheter for dialysis. However, by the time they got around to it, my father was decompensating and during the procedure for the arterial line, went into cardiac arrest.

He first coded when I was out on a walk trying to calm myself down. I was so angry about how this whole situation was being handled that I was about to lose it on someone. I rushed back to see that they had revived him. When I approached the new doc about putting in a dialysis catheter, she felt that he wouldn't survive the procedure. She said, "He's too unstable now."

"Why the *hell* didn't they do all this long ago?!" I asked her.

She said, "I am sorry, I don't know why. But I will do everything I can." She did, but it was too late. He coded two more times later that night. On their third attempt to resuscitate him, they did CPR for over 45 minutes. The doctor made eye contact with me, and I knew what that meant. I knew he wasn't coming back. I gave her the signal to stop, the hardest decision I have ever had to make in my life. After 45 minutes of CPR and 3 resuscitation attempts, he would likely have brain damage beyond repair. Just after midnight my father was gone. I watched his heart take its last beat and I literally collapsed into the doctor's arms. This is something I never want you to have to witness with your family members.

My dad went to the hospital to get the help he needed. But due to negligence and blatant carelessness, his health quickly deteriorated and in less than 30 hours he was gone. This was not an 80 year-old man! This was a 62 year-old man with life left to live! He had a perfectly treatable condition, pneumonia, that spiraled out of control because he was not properly monitored or cared for by medical staff.

I wish I had been there from the beginning because I would have asked the right questions and demanded medical attention for my father. My stepmom did not know what to ask or even what to do in that situation yet didn't ask for my help. Had I been there to keep tabs on the doctors and hold them accountable for their jobs, my dad probably would have survived his hospital stay. *His death was entirely preventable.*

A recent PubMed article estimates that medical errors are responsible for at least 251,000 deaths *annually* in the United States. After cancer and cardiovascular disease, it is the third leading cause of death in the US. Knowing that not all medical errors are reported, this number could be much higher. Other developed countries like Canada, Germany, and the UK have far fewer deaths from medical errors. So, what's the deal with the United States? Why are these mistakes all too common?

The answer to this question is my inspiration for authoring this book. The story I shared was one of the most awful experiences of my life. I don't want you to suffer through that kind of trauma like I did, watching my dad die needlessly at the hands of careless and negligent people... an experience that has changed my life forever. It is my goal to educate you about the state of our healthcare system so you don't end up there.

CHAPTER 1

OUR FLAWED MEDICAL SYSTEM

I have seen all too well how flawed our medical system is from the inside. Instead of educating people about nutrition, hydration, and a healthy lifestyle, we are over- medicating and under-investigating. Finding the root cause is the only way to fix the problem. Prescription medication is a band-aid that often relieves the symptoms, but not the problem itself and tends to cause more problems with its side effects.

I have witnessed a lot of mistakes by doctors and a ton of injustices on the part of insurance companies. Preventative tests or procedures get denied to patients who later end up in my emergency room with a life-threatening condition. Insurance companies want to save all the money they can, oftentimes at your expense.

Over the course of my career, I have come back to the same realization time and again: The root of the problem with our medical system is healthcare for *profit*. Medicine is a business, and like any other successful business, they care about increasing their profits and decreasing their expenses. The problem with this is that you, my friend, are the expense. Your health is the expense.

Most doctors enter the medical field with the primary intention of helping people. However, new doctors soon realize that their performance is heavily weighted on how much money they bring into the clinic or hospital. They are encouraged to see as many patients as possible in a short amount of time. Indeed, their jobs depend on it. I have witnessed this myself. Hospitals have a through-put algorithm to see how many patients an emergency room doctor sees in a specific amount of time. If they lag behind the average, they get "Talked To"! So, while they may want to give each patient the care and attention they deserve, their employer is cracking the whip to get the next patient in the door. Overloaded doctors and nurses tend to make more medical mistakes as they are pulled in a million different directions. Did you know most doctors are only allotted a 15-minute visit per patient *at the most*?

The recent pandemic was vital in exposing the healthcare inequality pervasive in the United States. Millions of employees were laid off during the shutdowns, leaving them without health insurance. If they were unlucky enough to get COVID, they had to pay for all expenses out of pocket. Luckily for some, during the beginning of the pandemic, the government picked up some of those expenses.

A lot of nurses contracted COVID working in the hospitals at the beginning of the outbreak. They didn't have proper personal protective equipment (PPE) for months, so nurses would often get huge viral loads from patients. Some of them died, and quite a few others were out of work for months recovering. Many nurses have been unable to return to the field due to long-lasting COVID symptoms.

Even though hospitals received huge stipends of money from the government during COVID to give their employees sick pay, some never saw a dime from their companies. I, myself, contracted a long-form of COVID and, while recovering, I certainly didn't see anything from HCA (Healthcare Corporations of America)! I used up all my paid time off and my extended leave, and then almost completely drained my savings account to pay out of pocket for the rest of the time off I needed to recover. Where did the money go that was meant to help people like me? The hospitals pocketed it!

Many other nurses went through this experience as well. Being denied COVID pay when they got the virus, they were left feeling unprotected and unappreciated. COVID took its toll on the nursing community. Not just physically, but emotionally. I saw more deaths in the first 8 months of COVID than I did in my entire emergency room nursing career.

Nurses are tough, but we are also human and can

only take so much. One in three nurses are now leaving the field entirely, claiming burnout after this incredibly demanding and hellish time.

Even though demand was up for nursing staff, hours were actually cut for some nurses. Some were put on furlough because they worked exclusively in surgery centers and were not trained for the hospital environment, while others saw a drop in their salaries.

The reason? Large corporate medical groups experienced a huge decrease in profits as non-urgent procedures were canceled because all hands were on the COVID deck. Treating COVID patients often meant long hospital stays and lots of resources utilized, directly resulting in less profit for the corporations. Their solution? Cut pay and cut staffing. This left the nurses who were still working in a state of exhaustion as they had to work long hours with limited staff and insane nurse-to-patient ratios. Vacation time? Forget it! The cold truth about how the medical system treats its employees came to the forefront of our minds. Medical workers blatantly saw how hospitals prioritized their bottom line over their staff. For many, it was the last straw that made them leave the medical field. While most of the public was sitting at home, medical staff were getting worked to the bone and getting sick with COVID.

For those of us nurses who still wanted to help people but also wanted to get treated well and paid what we are worth, a new opportunity was on the rise: Travel

Nursing. These two words have completely changed the lives and income of many nurses. With the high demand for emergency room nurses, hospitals started hiring independent contractors to fill in the gaps. Travel nursing is contract-based work, allowing nurses to pick and choose which contracts they take. The contracts vary between 4 weeks to a year but are typically about 3 months long. The pay is a lot higher than being an employee of a medical corporation. And vacations? Take all the time off you want in between contracts! We are now in control of our schedule and our pay. It is truly the silver lining that came out of the pandemic as the flaws of healthcare for profit became all too apparent.

Medical corporations saw their attempt at saving money backfire on them as more of their employees left for contract-based work. Hospitals began having to pay more to hire nurses on contract. As word spread about how lucrative this path is, more nurses chose to leave their employers to become independent contractors. Because of these staffing trends, *hospitals started lobbying Congress to put a pay cap on travel nursing!* To compound the problem, the industry has seen less and less doctors and nurses entering the field at all.

The pandemic shone a bright light on the financial vulnerability of almost all of the population. About 10% of the US population (31 million people) did not have health insurance at all during 2020. If they had to be hospitalized, they were sent home with a bill that they would never be able to pay. Even the people who did have health insurance were often stuck with huge medical bills that put them in debilitating debt when they were admitted to the hospital with COVID. It would be easy to assume that such a wealthy nation like the United States could support its citizens during a pandemic, however because corporations prioritize profit over the patients, a world-wide pandemic did not change their behavior.

Although polls have shown that two-thirds of the US population is in favor of healthcare for all, this will never happen while politicians and lawmakers are letting medical lobbyists line their pockets. It's important that we support candidates who have a real desire to fix this problem and won't be swayed by big dollars from the health insurance companies and the pharmaceutical industry.

My goal with this book is to teach you how to question everything about healthcare. You will not get the information you need unless you ask the right questions. Also, you need to learn to think critically about your own care and take an active role in your health. You have to think about you and your doctor as a *team* trying to solve a problem. Being your own self-advocate in a healthcare system that's working against you at every turn is crucial in getting the care you deserve.

If you are still looking at the healthcare system through rose-colored glasses, this book will make you take them off. I have seen too much over my career to think that a for-profit healthcare system is beneficial to anyone except the super-rich. Healthcare for profit results in subpar care that leaves people sick and in debt. Although US citizens pay more for healthcare than any other developed nation, overall health outcomes rank in the bottom percentiles. We are not paying more money to get better; we are paying more money to get sicker. I recently heard a doctor tell their friend, "Want to live? Stay out of the hospitals." Aren't we supposed to go into the hospital to get better?

As your own self-advocate, you need to:

1. Understand the medical system so you know what pitfalls to avoid.
2. When you are speaking to a doctor, learn to ask deeper questions until you understand what's going on.
3. Push for diagnostic tests when the doctor is acting blasé or when the insurance company denies you.
4. Don't just follow orders, take the wheel on your health, and demand the care you need!
5. Take care of yourself! Be responsible for your own health!

I have become extremely passionate about educating people about the healthcare system and about their own self-care. By the time you are finished reading this book, it is my hope that you have a better understanding of the healthcare system, feel empowered to take your health into your own hands, and demand the care you deserve from your healthcare provider.

I will also illustrate through my stories and experiences why sometimes you need to call in backup from a trusted health advocate. Through my 16 years of experience in many areas of the medical field, the negligence from healthcare providers and the greed of the health insurance corporations that I have witnessed has caused tremendous suffering in my own family and the families of my patients. It has motivated me to help others avoid the pitfalls of modern healthcare in the US by writing this book.

CHAPTER 2

MEDICINE IS A BUSINESS NOT A CHARITY

Healthcare for profit. These 3 little words are the reason that half of all Americans are in debt, the reason over 20,000 Americans die of treatable illnesses every year, and the reason 30 million of our citizens don't even have insurance.

America has, by far, the most expensive healthcare system on the face of the earth. Data collected in 2019 by the Organization for Economic Cooperation and Development (OECD) showed that America spent $11,072 per capita (per person) on healthcare while the average developed country spent $5,496 per capita. America's national health spending was 17% of our GDP in 2019 while the average of other comparably wealthy countries was 8.6% of their GDP. This means that *the average US citizen spends twice the amount on healthcare as citizens of other developed nations.* And these numbers have only gone up since then.

Countries that are part of the OECD are democratic societies with free-market economies such as Germany, Switzerland, France, Canada, Japan, Australia, the UK, and 30 others. While we pay twice as much as these other wealthy countries for our healthcare, we experience worse health outcomes than many of them. Compared to the average OECD nation, we have shorter life expectancies, higher disability rates, higher rates of suicide, more preventable deaths, and a greater number of infant and maternal mortality rates.

To top it all off, *we are the only developed nation that does not provide healthcare to all of its citizens.* While other nations in the OECD have a variety of healthcare infrastructures, they all cover every citizen so that everyone has equal access to care. By contrast, 9.2% of America's population, or 29.6 million people, lacked health insurance coverage in 2019. This number greatly increased when many got laid off during the pandemic shutdowns of 2020.

The COVID-19 pandemic really highlighted the problems with the American healthcare system. Because most people get their health insurance through their job, when the first shutdown happened, 7.7 million people (about twice the population of Oklahoma) lost their insurance coverage along with their jobs within a 3-month period. Those who were unlucky enough to get a serious case of

COVID and had to be hospitalized often got sent home with a huge medical bill. People who didn't have insurance were expected to pay out of pocket, leaving some millions of dollars in debt after getting sick. Even those who did have insurance were stuck with enormous deductibles and co-pays. Talk about adding insult to injury.

Today in The United States, the healthcare industry is the #1 most profitable sector of our economy (20% of our GDP). UnitedHealth Group, America's largest health insurance provider, brought in $242.2 billion in revenue in 2019. Johnson & Johnson, America's largest pharmaceutical company raked in $82.05 billion during the same year. The country's largest hospital, the New York Presbyterian Hospital, clocked in at $5.6 billion in revenue during 2019.

As millions of Americans lost their jobs and health coverage along with losing family members and friends, a wave of grief and panic struck the nation. Not only was there an intense fear of getting seriously ill from COVID and possibly dying, but Americans also realized that being hospitalized for COVID could result in going bankrupt and losing everything they had.

Meanwhile, health insurance and pharmaceutical companies were basking in the glory of sky-high profits from the pandemic. Health insurance companies thrived as elective surgeries and voluntary doctor visits were canceled. UnitedHealth Group saw a 44% increase in profits in the first quarter of 2021 compared to the year before. Insurers continued to rake in premiums while paying out less than ever before to healthcare providers. Do you think these companies paid it forward, helped with pandemic relief efforts, or gave any money back to their customers? Hell no! *But their shareholders sure were happy.*

Think about this, according to Open Secrets (a site that exposes who is lobbying Congress) Blue Cross/Blue Shield spent $25 *million* dollars of *your* hard-earned cash (and no doubt suffering) on lobbying members of Congress in 2021!

According to Forbes, Blue Cross revenues were $29 billion, that's right *billion*, and a net profit of $680 million in 2020, largely due to the fact that people were canceling their procedures because of the virus! They didn't suffer, they profited from COVID-19! Instead of passing that money back to the people, they pocketed it! That should be a crime! We could pay off half the US debt with just a few health insurance companies' revenues. Seriously think about that! While they are rolling in the dough, the average citizen has a life-altering medical bill to deal with.

Public funding of over $8 billion dollars (your tax dollars) to pharmaceutical companies Moderna, Pfizer, and BioNTech quickly got vaccines on the market. Fast forward to the height of vaccine distribution... These companies are making $93.5 *million* **per day** *in combined profits.* Despite these sickening profits, these companies refuse to distribute the vaccine or share their recipe with poor countries around the world, resulting in 98% of citizens in underprivileged countries being unvaccinated.

These massive monopolies own the patents to life-saving technology and use their power for profits, not for the good of humanity.

Pharmaceutical companies do this with all kinds of life-saving drugs, holding onto patents and setting astronomical prices on medicine only they can legally produce.

Remember Martin Shkreli? He took the drug called Daraprim from $13.50 per pill to $750.00 because he could! Although he did go to jail for only 7 years, the drug is still stupidly expensive. This has recently happened with insulin as well as epinephrine for allergic reactions!!! All for profit, literally on your life! Are you sick of it yet?!

Americans spend 10 times the amount on pharmaceuticals as citizens of other nations. For example, a $30 bottle of insulin in Germany would be around $300 in the United States. The US is one of Big Pharma's best customers, accounting for 48% of the global market and greatly contributing to its $1.27 trillion annual revenue (about $3,900 per person in the US). We are the only country in the developed world whose government imposes no restrictions on how much pharmaceutical companies can charge for their products. Trump had the best chance to make a change; he had the House, Congress, and the Senate. He talked big about doing it. But, it didn't happen. So, what happened to Trump care? Huge donations from Big Pharma and the Health industry, that's what happened! Big Pharma had policymakers wrapped around their finger, spending millions of dollars every year on lobbying Congress and the Senate so their prices remain unregulated. During the first 9 months of 2021, PhRMA (Pharmaceutical Research and Manufacturing of America) spent $23 million lobbying Congress. Pharmaceutical companies often claim their soaring prices are a result of research and development costs. However, a 2021 report released by the House Committee on Oversight and Reform found that 14 Pharmaceutical corporations spent $56 billion more on stock buybacks and dividends then they spent on research and development between 2016 and 2020. Clearly, these companies are working for their shareholders more than they are working for the American people, feeding us lies while they get filthy rich.

Another factor that makes our healthcare so expensive is that the US healthcare industry budgets 20% of its income for "administrative costs". This is at least *four times higher* than any other country. Administrative costs often equate to executive bonuses, larger dividends for shareholders, and huge salaries for those at the top. These costs are tacked onto the already high price tag of healthcare.

In the US healthcare is a luxury, not a right. Huge medical monopolies dominate hospitals, health insurance, and the pharmaceutical industry with little to no regulation from the government. Meanwhile, 500,000 Americans go bankrupt every year due to healthcare bills they can't afford. According to the American Journal of Public Health, 2 out of 3 bankruptcies in the US are tied to medical bills.

Our healthcare system is not broken, it is working exactly how it was intended to work by those who created it: corporations. Corporations identify a need in the market (healthcare), create a product to address the need (insurance, pharmaceuticals, hospitals), and market the product to make as much profit as possible. This is our free market economy at work. The difference between our healthcare system and that of other free-market economies? *We view healthcare as a business, not as a basic human right.*

There was recently an article on NBC news called "Private equity firms now control many hospitals, ERs, and nursing homes. Is it good for healthcare?" The article talks about how private equity firms are buying out hospitals and physician groups for profit. Dr. Lin was extremely concerned about his hospital's lack of preparedness for COVID. He went to his superiors regarding his concerns and got nothing from them. He turned to social media to express his concerns and was put on leave right away without review. He thought this was extreme and odd. Come to find out that his hospital had sold the ER doctors out to the private equity firm Blackstone Group (aka TeamHealth).

We have all heard about them. We might as well call them the evil empire. A private equity firm doesn't follow traditional hospital regulations. So, his right to due process disappeared, right along with lots of other patient safety regulations. Patient deaths in these private equity owned hospitals and nursing facilities have gone up substantially. This is due to their bottom line... profit over the patient. They cut staff, cut pay, invade the employee 401Ks and pensions, and find ways to cut every corner for profit. Again, you're a dollar bill....

So, how do you avoid a hospital or facility like this? Well, it may be harder as time goes along and Congress does nothing about it. These firms are buying facilities all over the place. They own about 25% of hospitals.

Apollo Global, overseen by Leon Black, owns RCCH (Healthcare Partners) and runs 114 hospitals. Cerberus Capital Management, run by Steve Feinberg, owns Steward Health Care; it runs 35 hospitals and a swath of urgent cares in 11 states. If you want to avoid these hospitals, find out who truly owns them and who owns the physician groups. Look for Carlyle Group (MedRisk), KKR & Co. (Envision Healthcare), Warburg Pincus (Modernizing Medicine), Apollo (Healthcare Partners), and Blackstone (Team Healthcare). These firms have spent BILLIONS to buy up facilities, gut them and make profit from them regardless of the human cost ($407 more per inpatient day [$407x5 day stay=$2,035]).

According to JAMA (Journal of the American Medical Association), in these private equity-run nursing homes, the chance of death goes up 10%. There are about 1,000 more deaths a year and patients are 50% more likely to be on antipsychotics. Mark Reiter is the residency program director of emergency medicine at Tennessee University and past president of the American Academy of Emergency Medicine. He says *"Private equity-backed healthcare has been a disaster for patients and doctors. Many decisions are made for what is going to maximize profits for the private equity company, rather than what's best for the patient and the community."*

Towards the end of 2020, a comprehensive multivariate analysis of factors affecting COVID infection and death in America was published by Families USA. This study found that having such a huge uninsured population actually increased cases of COVID-19. After controlling for a multitude of factors, researchers found that 44% of cases were associated with not having insurance.

Why? Uninsured people tend to delay care or forgo it completely due to the cost and end up spreading it to more people in their communities. Even more alarming, 32% of COVID deaths were linked to insurance gaps. This means that 1 in 3 COVID deaths was linked to health insurance gaps in the United States. When people can't afford care, they often do not seek it out, as they know the detrimental effect it will have on their finances. Many people waited until it was too late to go to the hospital. In a country as wealthy as the United States, this is unacceptable. Other developed nations take care of all their citizens at a fraction of the cost of what we spend on healthcare. It saddens and angers me that corporate greed left unchecked by the government has cost so many their health and their lives.

The question isn't, *"Can we afford to provide healthcare*

for all our citizens?" The real question is, *"Can we afford not to?"* The moral dilemma of healthcare for profit has stared us in the face year after year, yet our government turns its nose up at the idea that everybody deserves basic healthcare. *Funny, our Senators and Congresspeople get free top of the line healthcare...*

Those who don't want healthcare equality try to use the scare tactic that providing healthcare for all will turn the US into a socialist nation. We're not choosing between capitalism and socialism; we are choosing between profits and humanity. Every day we put a price tag on people's lives because of corporate greed, medical monopolies, and lack of government regulation or oversight.

But it wasn't always like this. Insurance companies and hospitals were at one time non-profits. The concept of insurance as we know it today was started in Dallas, Texas. In 1903, a 14-room hospital was opened called the Texas Baptist Memorial Sanitarium. Medical knowledge and treatments were improving at this time and many Texans came to be treated at this facility. Nobody was denied care and the hospital soon had many unpaid bills. To offset their losses, lawyer and vice president of the hospital, Justin Ford Kimball, offered an insurance plan to the local teacher's union. For $6/year, or $.50/month, teachers would be covered for up to 21 days of care in the hospital.

As word spread of this affordable insurance, more Texans wanted to purchase what they called "catastrophic care insurance". As medical advancements were being made, healthcare was becoming unaffordable to the average citizen, so health insurance presented a more affordable option. Between the late 1920s and the late 1930s, the new health insurance model spread throughout the country and by 1939, 3 million people had signed up. These "Blue Cross Plans" were not meant to make a profit, but to protect patients from draining their savings accounts in the event of illness. These plans were also meant to keep hospitals afloat along with the charitable religious groups that funded them.

During World War 2, Congress passed the stabilization act in 1942 which prevented employers from raising salaries in an attempt to stabilize the economy. This in part resulted in labor shortages and companies had a tough time attracting workers. In order to recruit more employees, companies started offering health insurance as part of employee compensation. Since insurance was not taxable and out-of-pocket healthcare was becoming more expensive, it was an enticing incentive that got people back to work. This was the beginning of the employer-sponsored healthcare that we know today.

Blue Cross and its partner Blue Shield were the major insurance providers at the time. Blue Cross covered hospital visits and Blue Shield covered doctor visits. Between 1940 and 1955, the percentage of Americans who had health insurance grew from 10% to 60%. Blue Cross/Blue Shield maintained its non-profit status, accepting anyone who signed up, regardless of age or health condition, and charged everyone the same rate. They became one of the most trusted brands in America at the time.

However, the growing demand for health insurance presents a business opportunity and soon, for-profit insurance companies came on the scene. These new companies were more selective about who they offered coverage to, accepting only young and healthy people who they could make profit from. They charged people differently based on age and had various plans for different amounts of coverage.

By 1951, for-profit insurers Aetna and Cigna were major players in the healthcare industry. Through aggressive marketing, these companies dominated the market through the '70s and '80s. Blue Cross/Blue Shield held to their mission to provide affordable care to all people but were losing money as they were still providing coverage to the sickest patients that the other insurers would not. In 1994, under great financial pressures, they threw in the towel on their charitable mission and became a for-profit insurer, gaining access to the stock market to quickly erase their deficits.

Nowadays, insurance companies make massive profits in a variety of ways. For one, they never pay doctors or hospitals for the entire amount that the services cost. They have an amount they pay for each service, regardless of what the doctor or the hospital charges. At the same time, they leave the rest of the bill for the patient to pay in the form of a co-pay or deductible. Sometimes the health insurance company refuses to pay any of the bill. Meanwhile, insurance companies charge extremely high premiums to patients month after month. The average health insurance premium for one person in 2020 was $448/month and for a family, it's $1,041/month.

Another sector of the healthcare industry that started with a pure mission but has morphed into a money-making machine is the hospital industry. In the 18th century, most families would call a doctor to come to their house when they were ill, paying the doctor at the time of service. Hospitals, then referred to as almshouses, were charitable organizations that housed the sick, poor, and destitute.

The two oldest hospitals in North America, the Charity Hospital in New Orleans and the Bellevue Hospital in New York opened their doors in 1736. These hospitals were seen as charity institutions, and they were a last resort for many. During the Civil War, army hospitals opened in every state in the Union to care for soldiers. After the Civil War, hospitals really started taking off as more people moved to cities and advancements in medical technology were taking place. Churches and local governments started to build more hospitals across the country. In 1873, there were 178 hospitals in the USA. By 1909, just 36 years later, there were 4,359!

In 1946, Congress passed the Hill-Burton Act which gave out $3.7 billion over the next 30 years for hospital expansion across the USA. When Medicare was signed into law in 1965, even more money was available for hospitals.

It's worth mentioning that when Medicare and Medicaid started, there were no for-profit hospitals. The first one opened in 1969. By 1975, America boasted 5,875 hospitals across the country. However, in the mid-'70s hospitals started to close. This was partially due to advancements in medical technology. People were able to be treated without a lengthy hospital stay. Mergers also played a role in the decreasing numbers. By 1983, 1 in 7 hospitals were for-profit, owned by investors who ran multi-hospital systems.

A huge wave of mergers and acquisitions occurred after the year 2000. In fact, between 2008 and 2014, there were over 750 of them. This trend is still going strong. As of 2019, 1,233 hospitals were investor owned (for-profit), a 63% increase from 1975. Hospitals went from being run as philanthropic institutions to being run as corporations.

As mergers happened, these companies got bigger and more powerful, letting them negotiate higher priced contracts with insurance companies. When hospitals are all bought up by one umbrella company, suddenly there is no competition, and these hospitals can charge what they want. At least 20% of hospitals are part of these monopolies. For-profit hospitals tend to position themselves in wealthy communities where their patients are likely to have top shelf private health insurance.

Meanwhile, hospitals that serve poor and rural communities are struggling to keep their doors open. Patients with less insurance coverage, Medicare, Medicaid, or no insurance at all come to these facilities. These hospitals don't turn anyone away and sometimes never get paid for their services. Also, the government pays about half of what these hospitals' standard fees are for Medicare and Medicaid patients, leaving them struggling to cover their costs. In desperate straits, these hospitals often get bought out by larger companies who raise their prices or eventually shut them down due to their lack of profit. This leaves underprivileged communities without close access to care.

Since hospitals know they will be paid a discounted rate from insurance companies and the government, they found a way to keep their profits high. Each hospital has what's called a Charge-master. This Charge-master is a document that lists the prices for all medical services and supplies, along with a billing code for each. What hospitals decided to do is set extremely high prices for everything so that when they were paid a discounted amount by insurance companies, they were still making huge profits.

The problem with this is patients who have no insurance or low coverage insurance get stuck with a highly inflated price for every service and medical supply they used during their stay.

In this billing system, everything is itemized and charged for. For example, being administered Tylenol in a hospital actually has three costs. A single Tylenol pill costs $15 and to have the nurse hand it to you is another $6.25. The plastic cup the pill comes in costs you $10. One pair of gloves is billed at $53. One alcohol swab used on the patient is $23. These are outrageous costs for such cheap items. Does this give you an idea of why more serious treatments are through the roof?

When you get a medical bill, **do not** *simply pay it!* Get an itemized bill and fight the charges that aren't legitimate. Hospitals have a charging system based on the severity of the injury and the extent of care you need. These services are charged a typical price categorized as level 1, 2, 3, 4, or 5. Many hospitals charge a level or two higher than the care you actually got. Hence, you could be paying thousands and thousands of dollars more than the care and treatment you received. All hospitals are required by law to post their costs. When you end up in the hospital, demand to see a charge sheet before receiving care, if it is possible.

When Bernie Sanders, our most recent political advocate for "Medicare for all", asked people in a Twitter post what the most absurd medical bills they had received were, horrifying stories started pouring in. $11,000 after having an allergic reaction and staying overnight in the hospital. $16,000 to diagnose a kidney stone. A $480,000 bill for spinal fusion surgery. $15,000 for an emergency c-section that the insurance company wouldn't cover. $120,000 per chemotherapy treatment. Does this sound like affordable healthcare to you?!

In life-or-death situations, people will pay whatever it costs to keep themselves or a loved one alive, and hospitals know this. They are fully aware they can get away with whatever ridiculous price they charge because they are the ones with the power to save your life. Hospitals, insurance companies, and pharmaceutical companies use our desperation to their advantage. At the very worst times in our lives when we are the sickest, medical corporations win big. *Greed, not goodwill, saturates every aspect of our healthcare system.*

I currently work with a doctor who is in a lawsuit against a county hospital. He tried to do the right thing, got pushed out and then blacklisted. It's a long story, but it is another example of greed and blatant disregard for patient safety. I cannot go into much detail because it is a pending lawsuit at the time of this writing. But the gist is, he was working for a hospital and found out that the CEO started to force physicians to send out patient results for things like ultrasounds, C.T. scans, and other important patient information to outside sources (telemedicine) to be read and reviewed. These outside sources were connected directly to her financially. This was pure profit, which costs the patient more along with losing time waiting for a reading. No one knew who these telemedicine doctors were, how reliable they were, and what kind of credentials they had. Watch for the story, he is trying to get it out there.

Health insurance companies, doctors, and pharmaceutical companies make more money when you are sick. It's the blatant and painful truth of the matter. I am convinced that this is the reason doctors do not get even one semester of nutrition education while the rest of their training focuses on pharmacology and surgery.

Guess who pads the back pockets of the medical colleges? BIG Pharma! They drive the syllabuses! According to a survey done by NPR, up to 16% of medical schools' yearly budgets are funded by the pharmaceutical industry.

As paradoxical as it seems, the healthcare industry does not profit off of you being healthy. They make the most money when you are extremely sick. This is why it is hard to find doctors who try to offer cheap and natural solutions before prescribing medication. It's important to remember this fact when taking advice from anyone in the medical industry. Always do your research and ask questions. A sick patient is a return customer. A healthy one is not.

Doctors and insurance companies should work hand in hand; however, doctors often get the shaft from insurance providers. They regularly find themselves in a tug of war for reimbursement, losing time and money submitting, disputing, and collecting claims. The American Medical Association estimates that 10-14% of a doctor's revenue is wasted on claims processing. (Also, hospitals across the country lose $262 billion every year from denied insurance claims.) Doctors and hospitals are trying to save lives while insurance companies are trying to make money. See the conflict of interest? Many people are reconsidering becoming doctors now. We already have a shortage of healthcare professionals; it's just going to get worse. Soon we will be in a major crisis. You think it's hard to get into a doctor now, just wait.

Doctors do, however, work hand in hand with pharmaceutical companies. Pharmaceutical reps are notorious for wine-ing and dining doctors, paying for their continuing education, giving them free travel, and offering other incentives that will encourage doctors to prescribe their pharmaceuticals.

A study published in The New England Journal of Medicine found that 94% of doctors admitted to having some sort of relationship with the pharmaceutical industry. With insurance companies being so stingy on one side, the overly generous nature of pharmaceutical companies on the other side is a strong temptation for doctors. This doctor-pharma relationship has played a key role in the opioid crisis, causing patients to be hooked on opioids for life as doctors keep refilling their prescriptions.

So, let's take an assessment of what we have here:

- Your insurance company will gladly take your money every month but keeps a tight grip on the money it will pay out to healthcare providers for your medical needs, often leaving you with large medical bills.

- Hospitals have Charge-masters that set ghastly prices for their services so they can keep increasing their profits even if private and public insurers pay them less than their standard fee for service. Those with no insurance or poor insurance will be charged the full price.

- Doctors get pressure from the corporations they work for to see more patients in a shorter period of time to increase profits. This results in a decrease in the quality of care and an increase in medical errors.

- A few doctors even pad their pockets with bribe money from pharmaceutical companies to push more pills onto you, the patient, who may or may not actually need them.

- Meanwhile, the government looks the other way during all of these injustices while accepting huge checks from Big Pharma and Insurance companies! The healthcare industry spends far more money on lobbying than anyone else, even the oil industry! Everyone gets rich except for you.

So, tell me, in this equation, who is looking out for *your best* interests? The sad and scary truth? Nobody is. And this is exactly why you need to educate yourself, learn to be your own advocate, and if necessary, seek help from a trusted health advocate.

CHAPTER 3

COMPARING HEALTHCARE NOTES WITH OTHER COUNTRIES

> "A nation as prosperous and successful as ours must guarantee the health of all its people. Safeguarding healthcare for every American is not a sentimental wish, it's a matter of justice."
>
> —Woodrow Wilson in 1912

For more than 100 years, many of our nation's leaders have advocated for healthcare equality in our country. However, a powerful group known as the American Medical Association along with many special interest groups have successfully opposed all attempts to provide healthcare for all. As a result, 22,000 Americans die every year of treatable diseases because they cannot afford healthcare.

The main difference between America's healthcare system and those of other countries is that we view healthcare as a business, not a basic human right. Advanced, industrialized, free-market democracies like our own provide healthcare for everybody and spend half as much as we do for it. In fact, America is the _only one_ of the OECD countries that doesn't have a system in place to provide healthcare for everyone. The reason these other countries make it work is because of their important upheld belief that medical care is a basic human right.

In America, our first question is always "How much will it cost?" instead of "How can we provide care for everyone?" Our fundamental idea that healthcare is a luxury, not a right, creates vast inequalities within our system. Those who can afford it get great care, but tens of millions cannot and do not. We have more uninsured people (31 million) than any other developed nation, and 25% of those who are well insured _still_ have trouble paying their medical bills! According to Credit Karma, 20 million of its members have $45 million of medical debt in collections... and that's just its members!

Imagine living in a place where an affordable healthcare premium is automatically deducted from your income, and you have insurance that pays every one of your claims in a short amount of time. Imagine having access to any doctor you wanted, and nobody is out of network because you're in a system that is all part of the same network. Imagine nobody becoming indebted due to medical bills if they get sick or have an accident. It sounds too good to be true, but it's actually how most other developed countries operate.

Take Japan for example. They have the longest healthy life expectancy while spending half of what America does on healthcare per person. There is an individual mandate which requires everyone to have insurance. With hundreds of insurance companies to choose from, competition drives prices down and this has created a system affordable for the Japanese. In fact, it is so affordable that the average Japanese person goes to the doctor around 15 times per year! People can afford preventative care and they definitely take advantage of it. Hospital stays are so cheap that most mothers spend 8-10 days in the hospital after giving birth. As a result, Japan has one of the lowest infant mortality rates in the world (⅓ the amount of America)!

Britain's National Health Service (NHS) is considered by experts around the world as one of the most cost-effective healthcare plans in existence. Brits pay nothing at the point of service and receive no medical bill. There is no co-pay, no premium, no fee at all. Since most people are eligible to waive the prescription fee, 85% of drugs in Britain are dispensed for free. Hospitals are government-owned, and many doctors are government employees. There is one insurance plan that covers everyone—the NHS! The NHS is a point of pride for citizens because it makes them feel a sense of solidarity that every citizen is taken care of no matter what their condition.

Germany is a country that chooses to keep healthcare privatized while fixing prices for its non-profit health insurance companies. These "sickness funds" are required to accept everybody and pay all claims. Germans have over 200 private insurance companies to choose from. If someone does not like their coverage, they can drop it and pick a new one for the same price. Sickness funds are offered through employment, with the employer paying part of the premium, and the employee paying the other part. If someone does not have employment or is transitioning jobs, the government pays the employer's part of the premium. Germans are covered by private healthcare from cradle to grave with no interruptions.

I recently flew with a gentleman that had an injury here in the states at work. He flew to Germany to see family and realized that his knee was worse than expected. He went to an orthopedic clinic for care and even though this was an injury that happened on the job in the states, he got amazing care. When he told them what happened and that he did not have German insurance, they said, "No worries, we got your back. It will probably be about 200 euros. We can get you in, in about 15 minutes, to see the doctor."

The doc came out and called the man in himself, evaluated him, drained his knee, did an ultrasound, did collagen and stem cells injections, told him to come back again in 2 weeks for a third injection, and gave him a brace. He had a meniscus tear and an MCL strain. When he went to check out and pay, he expected to have to pay an arm and a leg, possibly a kidney. The cost… 162 euros (equivalent to $165 US dollars at the time of this writing)! That was IT! On top of the amazing experience he had, his knee was even better than before the injury, avoiding an almost guaranteed surgery here in the states! ARE YOU SICK OF AMERICAN MEDICINE YET?

In America we are convinced that free enterprise creates the best product, but in healthcare, this proves not so. Other countries around the globe all agree that healthcare and profit do not go together. It is contradictory by nature to try to make a profit off sick people, but in the US it's the biggest sector of our economy in the for-profit arena. Our system favors the rich and excludes the middle class, leaving tens of millions out of the equation altogether… and it's only getting worse.

The main differences between America's healthcare system and those in other developed nations are:

- Governments in other countries regulate the medical industry to keep prices low for the patient.
- Insurance companies in other countries are non-profit organizations, instead of for-profit corporations selling shares on Wall Street.
- Other countries have an individual mandate requiring all citizens to be enrolled in some form

of insurance plan. This allows funding for public healthcare and ensures the patient access to get the care they need in any health situation they may face.

- In some countries, medicine is government run. In others, it is privately run with government regulation. In either case, the government plays a role in keeping costs down for drugs and services. In America, no price-setting or regulation happens from the government to the insurance or drug companies.

- In other countries, insurance companies cannot deny you coverage based on pre-existing conditions and cannot deny claims submitted for care. These foreign insurance companies pay for every medical bill submitted in less than a month (often less than a week). In America, insurance companies can legally refuse to pay your submitted medical claims and can even deny you coverage entirely.

- America had 31 million uninsured citizens in 2021. COVID has brought to light our system's weaknesses in terms of no job/no coverage. Through the pandemic, other countries still covered everyone through their individual mandates, taxation policies, and government subsidies.

- People in other developed nations are shocked by how much we pay for basic things like inhalers, insulin, epi-pens, even just an ambulance ride, which is free in most other countries.

- Part of America's excessive cost for healthcare comes from its 20% administrative budget (the largest of any country in the world). Most countries keep their administrative costs below 5% of their budget. This large budget pays for complicated billing and paperwork associated with this convoluted system. This large budget also pays for huge executive salaries and congressional "donations" (aka bribes).

- America is a nation that can afford to provide care for everyone but chooses not to.

- For this reason, people who can afford the best get the best. On the other end of the spectrum, there are those who have no insurance and can only get free help in a life-or-death emergency situation.

We know our healthcare system is not working for a huge majority of people. So why don't we change it? We have adopted many elements of other cultures into our own, such as interstate freeways from Germany, yoga from India, and pizza from Italy. So, what about healthcare? Why can't we look to other countries who are doing it better and cheaper and see what we can implement?

Let's learn about the four main health care models around the world:

National Health Insurance Model

- A government-run insurance plan that everyone pays into
- The government pays private doctors and hospitals to provide care for patients
- Since the government is the only purchaser of healthcare, they are able to negotiate low prices with pharmaceutical companies and hospitals/doctors
- There may be longer wait times for elective surgeries, but everyone gets acute care during a medical emergency or health crisis
- Canada, Australia, South Korea, Taiwan, Mexico

Beveridge Model

- Single payer government run national health service
- Healthcare is funded by the government through taxes
- Many medical clinics and hospitals are government owned
- Some doctors are government employees, others run a private practice and get paid by the government
- Government controls what doctors can do and how much they can charge

- No one ever gets a medical bill or has to pay anything out of pocket
- Great Britain, Spain, Scandinavia, New Zealand, Hong Kong

Bismarck Model

- Private doctors, hospitals, pharmaceutical companies, and insurance companies
- Everyone stays with private healthcare from cradle to grave
- Insurance companies are non-profit organizations
- An insurance company cannot deny anyone coverage, can't deny claims, and must pay claims within a short period of time
- People share the cost of health insurance premiums with employers
- If you lose your job, you still have insurance. Government acts as the employer and pays their share of the premium. If you can't afford any of your premium, the government will pay it all
- Germany, France, Switzerland, Japan

Out of Pocket Model

- Typically found in poor countries with no healthcare system

- Over 150 countries around the world use this model
- Pay per visit
- Pay with money or trade goods/services for treatment

Developed countries often use a hybrid model where the government runs the basic healthcare system, but private insurance companies offer supplemental care for better, faster services and amenities. The difference between them and us is they find a way to cover the basics for everybody while providing additional insurance for those who want extra and can afford it. America fails to offer even basic coverage to all of its citizens.

These 4 models of healthcare aren't just found internationally, they are all found in America as well. The US has all 4 of these models available to certain groups, but not one model available to all:

- The Veterans Health Administration represents the "Beveridge Model" of healthcare systems—government owned facilities and doctors funded by taxes
- When a working person splits their premium with an employer this is the Bismarck Model
- Medicare is the National Health Insurance Model—government insurance plan guaranteed to all over 65

- People who cannot afford insurance use the out-of-pocket model much like citizens of poor third world countries do. 31 million people (about the population of California) will have to pay out of pocket if they need any health care—medical bills that could be in the hundreds to millions of dollars.

Although some individuals (such as seniors and veterans) are taken care of by the government, and some jobs offer good healthcare, there is still a big gap of people who do not have access to affordable insurance. Some people get coverage through work while others are independent contractors who cannot afford big premiums and go uncovered.

People living well below the poverty line get Medicaid, but if you make slightly too much for Medicaid and are still too poor to afford health insurance, you must pay out of pocket as well. I personally am in that niche. I am a contract 1099 nurse. I make too much to get Medicaid, but not enough to afford good insurance. They want me to pay $500.00 a month for 70/30% with a deductible of $8,000 for the very basic level of insurance. Which quite honestly is SHIT! So, I only have emergency insurance. I am lucky to be very healthy and take extremely good care of myself. I am highly active, but do not take any chances to reduce the risk of injury. I am a Nurse and cannot get good insurance. IT SUCKS!!

We need a system that is all inclusive. We need a system that makes coverage affordable and available to all people, rich and poor, as we see in developed countries globally. If part of our income and/or sales tax was designated to fund a healthcare system for all, we could include everyone. People would end up paying less for this new healthcare tax than they do for their monthly premium *and* not worry about being denied care or being able to afford it. Culturally we would need a mindset shift that looks for solutions that include every person, not just the privileged.

Part of the slow change comes from special interest groups blocking all attempts to reform healthcare. America's government has been in the back pocket of pharmaceutical and insurance giants for decades now. Our lawmakers accept election donations from these mega corporations who have every interest in keeping things the same in healthcare, with little regulation from Uncle Sam. Until we hold our government accountable for implementing some guidelines on what insurance companies can and can't do, the average citizen will continue to pay the price.

Having everybody in the same system is fairer as everyone gets the same treatment when they are sick. Through these unified systems, some countries even use health cards (similar in looks to a credit card) that store a person's digital medical records in one place. Having everybody in one system means one set of rules, forms, and prices, which makes things vastly simpler, greatly cutting down on administrative costs and saving hundreds of millions of dollars. In countries where people are taken care of by a government-controlled healthcare system throughout their lives, there is more focus on preventative care which saves the system money in the long run.

1. **France:** Known for its Carte Vitale, a card that contains a chip with your entire medical history on it, France has what is considered one the most organized and effective healthcare systems in the world. France is characterized by universal healthcare and ranks high in health outcomes, accessibility, and advancements in medical technology.

2. **Italy:** Residents and legal immigrants receive primary care, preventative screenings, specialty care, maternity care, hospice care, inpatient care, and pharmaceuticals—all for free! No one pays a deductible and very few visits require a co-pay. Their National Health Service is funded through corporate and value-added tax revenues collected by the central government.

3. **San Marino:** Consistently ranked in the top three European healthcare systems, San Marino has universal healthcare. For those who work, a discounted premium is deducted from their pay. Self-employed people pay their own affordable premium. For the unemployed, aged, and other

vulnerable populations, healthcare is provided free of charge.

4. **Andorra:** With affordable premiums shared with employers, citizens of Andorra enjoy having 90% of hospital stays covered, 100% of maternity fees covered, and 75% coverage for specialists. The Lancet's Healthcare Access and Quality Index showed Andorra with the highest rankings.

5. **Malta:** Much like Britain, Malta has a long history of publicly funded healthcare for everyone. No one pays at the time of service or gets a medical bill.

6. **Singapore:** Three health insurance systems ultimately cover everyone. Through taxation, these three savings plans are big enough pots to help anyone in need. One fund is essentially a long-term savings plan for catastrophes, another is for routine expenses, and a third is for the underprivileged.

7. **Spain:** Not only do Spain's citizens get access to free healthcare, so do its migrants, regardless of legal status in the country. Anyone living in or traveling through the country won't have to worry about a medical bill while getting top of the line care.

8. **Oman:** Oman's government made a commitment to provide universal healthcare for the well-being of all its citizens, and it has done just that. With

help from oil and gas export revenues, the government has been able to build hospitals and employ doctors so that every person receives free primary care.

9. **Austria:** Austria's hybrid system has produced tremendous outcomes for the people living there. While all citizens are covered through the publicly funded health insurance system, many choose to get private supplemental coverage as well. Austrians enjoy close access to a variety of hospitals and clinics along with the lowest pharmaceutical prices in Europe!

10. **Japan:** The Japanese preventative approach to healthcare has resulted in a country with the longest life expectancy in the world. Affordable coverage is purchased through either the Social Health Insurance system (if you are a full- time employee) or through Japan National Health Insurance (if you are an independent contractor). Around 5% is deducted from wages of full-time workers to fund the country's Social Health Insurance system. Japanese citizens pay less than half of what Americans do for superior healthcare.

A few common threads are woven throughout the countries with the highest healthcare rankings in the world. First, the government makes a commitment to its people to provide basic health coverage for everybody, whether people can afford it or not.

Second, hospitals and health insurance companies in these countries are operated as non-profit organizations with the goal of providing healthcare for everybody. This means no denying patients based on pre-existing conditions and no denying medical claims.

Third, the government plays a crucial role in the healthcare system, regulating prices and policies so that everyone gets fair treatment and affordable healthcare.

America has so much to learn from other countries that are doing healthcare better, cheaper, and more efficiently. We've got to be able to recognize that our way is not the best way, and millions are suffering because of this.

It all must start with a commitment from our government that every citizen *does* deserve healthcare. No one living in the US, one of the richest nations in the world, should be turned away because they cannot afford care. Countries with universal healthcare make the decision that there is enough to go around. When the vast majority of citizens are paying into the system, the vulnerable populations can be covered too, and everyone can enjoy equal access to the care they need. Keep your eyes peeled for candidates who understand the importance of this topic and are willing to make substantial changes to our healthcare system so that everyone can finally be included. Remember, your health depends on the health of others. Would you want someone making your meal that has hepatitis A and cannot get care? Or someone that is coughing up blood, but doesn't go to the hospital or doctor because of the exorbitant cost? That could be tuberculosis (contagious)…everyone matters!

You may wonder why I am expressing the importance of this subject of healthcare and how it involves self-advocacy. You can change this by voting the right people in and demanding change! In my opinion, the only other way we can force the change is if EVERYONE STOPS PAYING FOR HEALTH INSURANCE, even corporations that provide it to their employees. The system will collapse within the month forcing healthcare for all. An example of this is Martin Luther King trauma center. They closed due to the inability of the people to pay their medical bills. We have had many trauma centers close due to this. As the population grows, we need more trauma centers, not less. The same thing will happen to the big health corporations if we stop pouring money into their pockets.

Therefore, I stress the importance of voting the right people in. Neither Republican nor Democrat have any interest in healthcare for all. They make too much money to vote otherwise. You can find out who votes which way by paying attention to what's on the docket and how your representatives voted. You cannot just vote someone in and then go about your life, you must pay attention. So far, it seems only the progressives and independents have voted for some form of healthcare for all. You want change, become an active participant in our system and pressure your representatives.

In the rest of this book, I will explain how to be your own self-advocate in the system we are in now. BUCKLE UP! Here we go!

CHAPTER 4

WHAT YOU DON'T KNOW CAN KILL YOU

What you don't know can kill you, and for many people it has. Working as a Registered Nurse in the emergency room for 12 years has made this enormously apparent to me.

Most people have no idea what questions to ask their doctors and nurses to ensure they are getting the proper care. Heck, most people don't even know what their prescription medication is called, and they wouldn't be able to tell you to save their lives.

The problem lies in an education barrier between the medical staff and the patients. Due to the fact that doctors have much more education than the average patient, patients put full faith in their doctors and often trust them with their lives, a mistake that can have deadly results.

What my stepdad didn't know almost killed him. He

was having pain radiating down his arm, tightness in his chest, with a little shortness of breath. I told him to go to the emergency room immediately. He was monitored for a short time, got lab work and an ECG done, which seemed to be normal. I told my mother to NOT LET THEM SEND HIM HOME! I sternly told my mom to demand they hold him overnight for observation and get a stress test before releasing him. Luckily, he had a talented team who agreed to hold him in the hospital.

It's a damn good thing they did, too, because the next day during a stress test my stepdad had a massive heart attack. It was discovered that he had a 99% blockage in his LAD (the main artery behind his heart), what we call in the ER a "widow maker". If he had not been so close to emergency medical care, he most likely would have died before getting to the hospital.

Because I recognized the signs and symptoms of a heart attack, my stepdad was able to remain in a setting where he could be monitored and treated immediately for his heart attack. Some people ignore the signs or don't know what to look for, or even agree to be released from the hospital when they know there is still something wrong. Because of this, many don't make it through a massive heart attack like that.

I took care of a friend that came in for chest pain a couple of years back. The same thing happened to him... normal labs but his ECG looked kind of suspicious. The cardiologist on staff that day thought the ECG looked okay and said to discharge him and have him follow up with them at their office. I told my ER doc, "I know this guy, he doesn't look good, and that ECG doesn't look right to me." The Cath lab nurses agreed with me along with the ER doc. I told the doc, "Don't discharge him. Send him to the Cath lab for a diagnostic angiogram." We convinced the cardiologist to do so. Guess what? He had a 99% blockage of the LAD as well! Good nurses that are willing to stick their necks out for you are extremely valuable, and they are leaving the industry in droves!

A patient I recently saw in the emergency room did not get as lucky as my stepdad. His problem was not a clogged artery, but cancer. He had known something was wrong for months, telling his doctor that his leg hurt. Not having good insurance, his doctor didn't bother ordering any diagnostic tests like an MRI. One day he fell snowboarding and was brought into an ER. After running a few tests, they found out that he had stage 4 bone cancer. A condition that could have been successfully treated in earlier stages; his cancer was now a death sentence as it had spread throughout his body. Yet another example of "what you don't know can kill you".

The beauty of modern medicine is that we can catch diseases early on in their development and use the tools we have to treat them before they become life threatening. The problem in America is that 31 million people without insurance can't afford these expensive diagnostic tests out of pocket. An MRI without insurance is between $650 and

$2200 depending on where you go. A CT scan can put you out $910-$9000! Many people who have no insurance or poor insurance often don't receive help until their disease has progressed to a more serious stage.

Luckily, the Affordable Care Act has made medical coverage accessible and affordable to many more people than before. Insurance can no longer deny you based on your medical history or charge more for pre-existing conditions. Each state has its own healthcare marketplace where healthy competition drives premiums down. State governments decide how much of a subsidy each person is eligible for based on their income. With some simple research and filling out a few pieces of paperwork, you could get healthcare easier and cheaper than you think. This program would've been much better, like the ones you learned about in the last chapter, had politicians funded by bribes from Big Pharma and the health industry not torn it apart!

Regardless, if you get insurance through your work, through a state marketplace, or through government programs such as Medicaid, Medicare, and the VA, there are things you can do to stay knowledgeable about your health. Just as what you don't know can kill you, what you DO know can keep you alive.

Let's start with the basics:

> **Allergies.** Do you know all of your allergies? Have you ever had an allergy test? If you are someone who has ever had a

reaction to food or medicine, you may consider getting a full allergy panel done to determine if you are allergic to anything else. If you have a severe allergy, you can carry Benadryl and an Epi-pen with you to prevent anaphylaxis. Always carry a list of your allergies with you so in the event you are unconscious, your caretakers can be aware of them. Wear a band or a necklace if it's a common drug or food like peanuts. As an ex Firefighter/EMTII, there have been many scenes we rolled up on with unconscious patients. We may end up administering a drug to save your life that you may be allergic to. That could ultimately kill you.

What else is important to know?

Blood type- If you are suffering from extreme blood loss and need an emergent transfusion, knowing your blood type will save time in the emergency room, valuable time that could save your life. Write this on your information card with your allergies.

Family health history- If you don't know, ask around and dig into your family's medical past. There are diseases you may not know you have but have occurred throughout your family tree. Doctors and nurses will consider these as potential problems when trying to diagnose your medical condition so keep this on your card. You do not have to put all your family history. List the important ones, like heart conditions, cancers, diabetes, and strokes.

Medications- are another super important thing for you to know and be able to communicate with others. This is where you may have to get a little technical and learn some medical terminology. Learn the names and dosages of your medications (many people don't know the name but can tell you the color and shape which is **_not useful_**). Every drug maker makes the same drug in a different shape and color. When I was a firefighter, we happened to roll up on an accident and one of the people was acting drunk. We didn't smell alcohol on them, which we thought was odd. So, we searched their car and found a blood sugar monitor. They weren't drunk, they were having a diabetic crisis.

Past surgeries- are a good thing to know. We don't need to know that your wisdom teeth were pulled at 10. We want important surgeries, like appendectomy, kidney transplant, heart stents, bowel surgery. I had a patient come in with severe nausea and vomiting. They weren't oriented enough to tell us that they had a bowel resection a couple years ago, which would've been useful since that ultimately ended up being the problem.

We also need to know if you're a **DNR** (do not resuscitate), which means "do not do CPR". A folded copy of your advanced directive is a good idea as well. This is important because we have held patients in the ICU for days and sometimes weeks, because we have no information on them whatsoever.

Your medical conditions- this is the most important. Your medical history; diabetes, heart attacks, strokes, long COVID, cancer, dementia, etc.

Family contacts- extremely important and more than one is absolutely necessary. We have held people in the ICU for long periods of time because we have not

been able to get a hold of a family member.
If we never get a hold of one, they either
end up dying there or being transferred to
a nursing home and waste away.

On the following page, you will find an example of what you would write on a medical card that you should carry with you at all times. Yes, it means taking the time to do it. But your life may depend on it one day.

Full Name	Blood Type	Code Status: DNR/Resuscitate
Date of Birth	Date Updated	Family Members Name & #

Medication List

Medication Name	Dosage (mg)	Frequency	Prescribing Doctor
RX			
Include Herbs and Supplements			
Include over the counter medications			

Allergies (Drugs, Food, and Medical Equipment like Latex)

Allergy			
Reaction			

Medical History

Condition/ Diagnoses/ Surgeries	Date of Occurence	Currently Active or Resolved	Doctor/specialist that treated your condition + phone number

Family Health History

Family History of Disease	Which Diseases/ Which Family Members?	Did a family member die of the disease?

When you're putting together your survival guide, make sure that it can fit in your purse or wallet. Design it so that it is double sided to save space. It should be a quick reference guide and not something that the paramedics have to read in depth to get the important information. So, all the super important information should be on one side, and the in depth information that the emergency room nurse and doctor can use to help save your life on the back. The Paramedics want to know allergies, medical problems I.E. diabetes and heart conditions (not your life history of problems, the important ones), important medications you're on (not all the vitamins you take), phone numbers to contact in case of emergency, and whether or not you are a DNR. If you are a DNR, have that paperwork with the survival guide. Everything else should be on the back or below the quick reference information. The more information regarding your health that you can fit on this paper the better. The rest of the "what I call non important info" can be in detail on the back. Like, all your other medical problems, vitamins and over the counter medications you take, along with your family medical history etc. Now, I am not saying that this isn't important information, it is. It will be extremely valuable to the emergency room staff. But, it's not something the Paramedics necessarily care about for the short time you are with them. They are concerned with getting you alive to the ER. Generally, they don't have time to delve deep into your history. So, take the time to put this together.

This is a basic format to help guide you in that direction. Consider laminating it for protection.

So now that you "know thyself" and have a list of information in your pocket, what are some things that are important for you to know? How can you make sure you are getting all the care you deserve even though you never went to medical school and don't understand how every disease works in the body?

If you are trying to diagnose a health problem, and even if you are just getting routine checkups, getting blood work done is one of the quickest ways to see what's going on inside your body. This gives you an idea of what your hemoglobin (red blood cell) count is, what your cholesterol levels are, and if your blood sugar is within a normal range.

With various pieces of information from a blood panel, your doctor can start painting a picture of what's going on inside of you. Silent killers like high cholesterol and diabetes can be detected with a simple blood panel. Also, ask for a copy of your results so you can research your numbers yourself.

Another example of "what you don't know can kill you" - melanoma. This malignant skin discoloration can be diagnosed with a biopsy. Do a google search of melanoma images to get an idea of what to look for on yourself. If you have anything that meets the criteria of this disorder, you can demand a biopsy immediately. If you know what to look for in terms of other skin cancers, you can catch something early before it spreads to the rest of your body. By doing a weekly skin check on yourself in a full-length mirror, you can save your own life.

It is often difficult to detect when something is going on deep within the bones, muscles, and organs of the body. Yet if we are in tune with our bodies, often we get early warning signs about problems on the horizon. Sometimes it's a dull ache, a sharp pain, or something that just doesn't feel right. We need to trust our body's inner wisdom enough to know that when our body talks, we should listen. If something becomes a persistent and noticeable problem, do not hesitate to get the proper test, even if your doctor waves it off as a non-issue. **Trust yourself.**

But what test do you need for what condition and how do you know if you should demand a test or not? In diseases like cancer and serious conditions like internal bleeding, most of the time people don't even know it's there until it has progressed significantly. Consider these diagnostic tools if you think or have evidence that something is wrong in your body. (Most good doctors would order these as a next step in the diagnosis of a health problem. However, if you don't have good coverage or none at all, your doctor may not offer these to you voluntarily. In this case, ask specifically for them.)

CT Scan

Often used to assist surgeries, biopsies, and radiation therapy, here are a few other uses for a CT scan:

- Find internal bleeding and its source
- Detect the presence of cancer, liver masses, lung nodules, and heart disease
- Identify the location of a blood clot or tumor, such as a stroke
- Diagnose a bone or muscle disorder, such as a fracture or tumor

The patient I mentioned earlier with bone cancer that came to see me in the emergency room should have gotten a CT scan when he initially started feeling pain in his leg. It would have located the cancer in the leg and treatment could have started immediately. But because this was not done, the cancer was found in its later stages.

X-rays

When we think of getting an X-ray, most of us think of broken bones and fractures. But X-rays can detect a lot more including:

- Enlargement of the heart
- Foreign object swallowed or lodged in the body

- Digestive issues
- Cancers and tumors
- Osteoporosis
- Arthritis
- Tooth decay (cavities)

When a patient complains of pain in the muscles/joints/bones, usually an X-ray is the first test done to rule out a bone fracture or tumor. X-rays don't show details of ligaments, tendons, and muscles, which is why the next test is often an MRI or a CT scan.

MRI's

MRIs produce high resolution images that are often used to take a closer look at soft tissues and the nervous system. Instead of using damaging radiation to take images, MRIs use magnets and radio waves to create detailed images on a computer. They can detect issues such as:

- Brain Injury/Tumor
- Stroke
- Spinal Cord Injuries
- Eye Problems
- Heart disease
- Clogged blood vessels
- Problems with the aorta

- Pericarditis (inflammation of the tissues around the heart)
- Spinal disk problems
- Joint damage
- Arthritis
- Breast, Ovarian, Kidney, Liver, Prostate, and Pancreatic cancers
- Also used to identify and track tumor growth

Ultrasounds

Ultrasound uses sound waves to create a picture and can record video of organs in motion. Checking for breast cancer is actually safer with an ultrasound than it is with an X-ray due to the harmful radiation involved in getting an X-ray. (It's way more comfortable too, no more squished boobs.)

Ultrasounds show things in motion, such as blood pumping through vessels, a heart beating, and a baby moving.

A pregnancy ultrasound is used to determine information about the baby's health and development such as:

- What size the baby is and if there is more than one
- Estimate how long you have been pregnant
- Check for birth defects in the spinal cord, heart, brain, etc.
- See if there are signs of Down's Syndrome

- Check the position of the baby
- See how much amniotic fluid the baby is surrounded by

During a diagnostic ultrasound, the goal is different depending on the area:

- Check a breast lump to see if it is cancer
- Identify the cause of abnormal menstrual bleeding
- Find the source of pelvic pain
- Check for malignant and benign growths on the thyroid gland
- See if blood is flowing at a normal rate
- Check for abnormalities in the heart and abdomen
- Ultrasounds can also help guide biopsies to make sure the correct tissue sample is taken

Blood Work/labs

A blood draw is a great way for the docs to see how your body's organs are functioning. Through these numbers, they can usually get a diagnosis or a really good idea of what's going on. You can easily look them up on the internet, it's pretty general and involves a range of numbers which can be referred to. For example, low HGB (hemoglobin) values will indicate that you are anemic. Why you're anemic will have to be investigated further, but at least you have an idea of why you are feeling exhausted.

Go over these numbers with your doctor and do your own research. The range of conditions can be huge when it comes to abnormal labs. In the ER, it's usually the first thing we do with a sick patient. It's the best and quickest way to get an idea of what's going on. You can even get a blood draw to diagnose certain cancers.

These are all tests that help doctors see inside your body to determine where the source of the problem is. The sooner the problem is found, the quicker a treatment plan can be put in place. The key is to make sure you are getting the problem identified as soon as possible.

Pop-up testing facilities are becoming more popular, offering patients ultrasound services for a minimal cash fee. These traveling testing sites allow people to take control of their health without waiting for a doctor's referral or an appointment. You can find out if there are blockages in your arteries, if you have breast cancer, and other pressing concerns.

Preventative testing is often covered by health insurance, and you should not hesitate to get these done… tests like a colonoscopy to check for colon cancer or other bowel issues. A pap smear can diagnose all kinds of disorders, from STIs to cervical cancers. A simple skin check from your primary doctor can identify potential skin cancers. Your health matters and by taking advantage of modern medical technology and advanced testing (heck even just having your doctor look you over), you can save yourself from suffering in the long run.

As most developed countries have realized, an ounce of prevention is worth a ton of treatment. Educating ourselves about how the body works and learning to recognize signs and symptoms of disease can help catch things early on. Keeping up with our preventative screenings can help catch diseases in their early stages. We are the gatekeepers of our bodies and must keep watch of what is happening within as well as without.

Remember, what you don't know can kill you, but what you *DO* know can save your life.

CHAPTER 5

DOCTOR DEATH

All of us nurses knew him by the same name… Doctor Death.

We all had our stories about him: who he killed on accident that week and which patient he gave the wrong medication to. He was the kind of doctor you hoped and prayed you or your family would never be under his "care". And yes, as nurses in a hospital system, we know which ones to avoid! We say, "Oh man! Don't EVER let that guy take care of me!!!"

Many times, I would catch him prescribing the wrong medication. When I would see his orders on the computer to give a certain medication, I was often confused as to why a medication that did not fit the patient's diagnosis was prescribed. Luckily, my years of training as a nurse, firefighter/paramedic, and advanced diver medic familiarized me with many medications. I was able to recognize what the medication was meant to do and what condition it treats. Because of this valuable knowledge, I saved some patients just by double-checking the prescription. When getting prescribed a new medication, ASK what the medication is for and about the potential side effects and contra-indications with other prescriptions you're on! It may save your life one day!

When I had an encounter with "Dr. Death" I called the doctor and asked him why he had prescribed this particular medication. "Oh, that was a mistake, that was for a different patient," he would say nonchalantly. *Well, it's good I caught it then, wasn't it?!* Many nurses would just administer whatever the doctor ordered, without questioning them. Some of this is a lack of knowledge, some is blind trust in the doctor, and often nurses just have too many patients to keep track of.

Everybody makes mistakes, sure, but there should be checks and balances in place. In a well-functioning system, everybody would double-check each other's work. But when doctors and nurses have too many patients, mistakes get overlooked in the frantic pace of the hospital setting. Doctor Death made multiple mistakes with multiple nurses. As all of us nurses started talking to each other, we realized that many of us had similar stories to share. Word was getting around about the dreaded Doctor Death.

One patient under his care was severely neglected and I had to fight for his right to get the treatment he needed. This was a patient with liver failure who was waiting to be transferred to USC for a liver transplant. He was not getting any fluids administered to him. I noticed that he had a super dry tongue and tenting skin. Although it was standard procedure to limit the amount of fluids given because fluids would likely be shunted to the abdomen, he very obviously needed *some* fluids.

This man's wife was getting concerned. She had been in and out of the hospital with her husband and had seen how negligent the doctors could be. Doctor Death was dismissive every time I called to update him on the patient's condition. After getting nowhere with the doctor, I advised the patient's wife to start talking to another doctor and get proactive about getting her husband transferred to USC for his surgery.

On top of letting this man get severely dehydrated, Doctor Death also wanted him on blood thinners. The thing with liver failure is, your blood is already having a tough time clotting, so adding a blood thinner on top of it could be detrimental, especially right before surgery. Understanding the severity of the consequences of administering this medicine, I refused to give it to the patient. After bringing it to the doctor's attention, I found out the prescription for this blood thinner was meant for another patient!

Doctor Death could have killed this patient in multiple ways, and if it wasn't for my diligence, along with getting another doctor involved in the case, the patient may not have made it to USC for the transplant. I filed a report about this incident as many other nurses had filed reports against him in the past about similar situations. Shortly after this particular incident, Doctor Death was no longer at the hospital. No one knew where he was or if he got fired.

A couple of months later, I ended up getting a letter from the hospital thanking me for filing the report against him. They claimed that I probably saved the patient's life by advocating for his care. I was surprised by this border-line admittance of fault regarding the doctor, and grateful I no longer had to work with him.

Happily, I didn't see Doctor Death for many years. I assumed he had gotten fired and maybe even had his license revoked. Management was always very secretive about cluing us nurses in. However, during the pandemic, I was doing contract work at various hospitals. One day I was in the cafeteria of a different hospital than I normally worked at and guess who walked up to order food…

You guessed it… Doctor Death. Even though he had multiple reports filed against him over many years, this negligent doctor was still allowed to practice medicine and have people's lives in his hands. Often doctors don't get fired, they are given the option to resign and then end up moving onto another hospital. This should show you how little accountability there is for doctors. Nurses are held to a much stricter standard, and often nurses become the scapegoats for doctors' mistakes, while doctors can literally get away with gross negligence. Another doc that

I worked with said this, "Do you know what a doctor who graduated with a "D" is called? DOCTOR!"

A most recent example of this was the nurse that worked for Vanderbilt Hospital, RaDonda Vaught. She was convicted of negligent homicide after ACCIDENTALLY giving the wrong drug to a patient that happened to die. There were multiple issues that the hospital was responsible for that led up to that final error, including the doctor. Were they held accountable? HELL NO! We can't have that exposed!

Nurses are expected to administer the right medications at the right times to the right patients. That means that even if the doctor orders the wrong medication, if I as a nurse give it to the patient and they have an adverse reaction, I could be held liable. That means I'm expected to research any medications that I don't know while taking care of multiple patients on multiple meds. Do you think nurses have time for this on top of all their other responsibilities? Heck no!!!

Have you ever wondered why the nurse never called you back? Or why they never have time to take a family member's call? Because we are running around managing 4 to 5 patients, their family members, and their doctors at a time with many responsibilities, little ancillary staff, managing changing patient conditions and emergencies, helping the CNAs with bed baths, trying to get a hold of doctors, AND documenting on all patients. These are just the basics. There are a lot more responsibilities than this that we are being held accountable for.

So, think about other states. They don't have nurse-to-patient ratios like California does. They could be taking care of 8 patients! The nurse's unions have been fighting to get a federal standard for nurse-to-patient ratios for years! Again, corporations' greed and lobbying take hold and it does not happen. This literally affects your standard of care in the hospital. In the end, it leads to lots of unnecessary deaths! You may be 1 of 8 patients one day. So, become proactive and call your representative to demand safer nurse-to-patient ratios.

The scary thing is that Doctor Death was not alone in his mistakes. Thousands of doctors prescribe the wrong medication, neglect their patients, and give them care that is often too little too late. **Researchers estimate that 250,000 to 440,000 deaths every year are attributed to preventable medical errors.** This is more lives than car accidents and gun violence take every year times 7! This has consistently been the 3rd leading cause of death in America for many years, only recently surpassed by COVID-19. When being given a drug, ask the nurse what the drug is for and if it is the appropriate dosage for your weight. Don't let them say, "oh yeah, it's fine". Make them show you in the pharmaceutical book of dosages.

I've had patients in the ER for 12 hours because there are no beds available in the main hospital. In some cases, the patient had not been seen or treated by an attending physician, even though they had been notified of the new patient and had transition orders from the emergency room doctor. There would be no food orders, no medication orders, nothing.

Often, I couldn't get in touch with these patients' doctors, and I would have to persistently call my house supervisor to try to help me locate them. These patients could need insulin or other life-saving medication. I would have no orders and no doctor to prescribe what the patient needed. This put an incredible amount of stress on me, having my hands tied, knowing what the patient needed, and not being able to do anything about it.

If you are ever in this situation, be kind to your nurse. In many cases, it's not their fault. Demand to see the charge nurse or the house supervisor. Oftentimes, your complaint will get better attention than the nurse's complaint in helping your case along. Please do not blame your nurse, thank them for trying and make sure the charge nurse understands that your complaint isn't against the nurse.

Sometimes, I would beg other doctors to help with my cases just to get the help my patients needed. Some would, some wouldn't. See, doctors are hesitant to take on patients that are not assigned to them because they don't want to be liable for treating another doctor's patient. In many ways, lawyers have destroyed this country (this is another story entirely). Even when these doctors could not be reached for a ridiculous amount of time, causing the patient an incredible amount of distress, they were never held accountable. They would get a slap on the wrist and be told not to do it again. What would happen? They would do it again.

Working in the hospital gets some of us nurses better treatment when we or our families need medical care. It's just an added benefit of knowing the staff personally. However, my nurse friend got the opposite of special treatment for her son.

She had brought him into the hospital that she worked at after he had his first seizure. After doing a few basic tests, the staff couldn't find anything unusual and insisted that he didn't have a seizure and released him. A few days later her son had a second seizure and had fallen in the shower and was now unconscious and seizing. The bathroom door was locked, so she and her husband had to break down the door to get to him. She called an ambulance and they took him to the emergency room.

By this time, *my friend was livid.* Instead of admitting her son for observation to find out why he was having seizures the first time, the hospital released him. Imagine if he had had a seizure while he was driving! He could have killed himself and countless others!

"This is the second seizure in a week! What is going on with my son?!" she exclaimed to the doctor.

"Well," her son's doctor replied sheepishly, "we missed something on the CT scan... Your son has a brain tumor."

"Really?! How did you miss that?!" She cried. "Didn't you even look at it?"

"Well, I didn't look at the CT scan myself, I was relying on the radiologist, and they didn't put a note in his file that anything was wrong."

"Really? They couldn't identify an obvious and visible brain tumor on the CT scan, for God's sake, I can see that!"

"Yeah… that was our mistake."

And again, this doctor was not held accountable for his mistake and is still working there. Sure, people can sue their doctor, but the doctor remains untouched as his malpractice insurance covers the bill and he continues to work without any consequence from the hospital or medical board. One doctor I work for said, "If there was a cap on malpractice insurance, doctors would be more careful with what they do. Less errors would occur."

I'd like to share my friend's story about an incident that affected her deeply in her career. She is also a nurse and was caring for a patient that had a DNR (do not resuscitate) order. Although they shouldn't, doctors often treat these patients more nonchalantly.

This patient was in her 80s which could have also contributed to the doctor's lack of motivation in keeping this woman alive.

My friend saw that this patient's kidney numbers were getting worse and worse. Her electrolytes were also imbalanced, and she was starting to show signs of kidney failure. My friend asked the attending doctor who was caring for the patient, "Shouldn't we get a nephrologist involved?"

"No," said the doctor, "I'm going to try a few things first."

Over the next 3 days, my friend saw this patient's health decline as their kidney function got significantly worse every day. She told the doctor multiple times that she strongly recommended getting a nephrologist (kidney specialist) involved in the case to help.

Multiple times, the doctor turned her down, saying he had other approaches to try.

When my friend saw a nephrologist in the hallway she told him, "I have a patient I really think needs your help."

"Do we have a consult yet?" he asked, meaning had the doctor put in the order for a specialist?

"No, but I really think you need to see this patient," she said adamantly.

"Well, we need to wait for a consult to be put in," he said resolutely. Rules are rules, right? Doctors won't cross the red tape, not even to save a life.

On the third day, my friend saw that the patient was declining rapidly, having multi-system organ failure originating from the issues in her kidneys. "So, when are we getting a nephrologist involved? Because what you are doing is clearly not working," my friend said to the doctor. The doctor didn't respond, and my friend went to lunch. When she got back, the patient was coding and died shortly thereafter. If this woman would have gotten the care she needed from a specialist, her life could have been saved. However, attending doctors know that they get paid a certain amount for each patient, and once they pass off their patient to a specialist, they get paid less.

Due to the pride, greed, and carelessness of the doctor, he would not ask for the specialist's help and allowed the patient to die needlessly. My friend was heartbroken.

When I have family in the hospital, I always ask to see their test results. I want to SEE the blood work numbers, I want to SEE the CT scan, I want to SEE it all with my own eyes. I don't trust the doctors to thoroughly review the test results, and since I know what to look for, I demand to see the results. A good doctor with nothing to hide will gladly show you the results. In fact, it is your legal right to have access to any and all test results. The good thing about this is, you both get to go over the results or images together. Have them explain it to you. Even if there is nothing there, if something had been missed, it would likely get caught during this time. Just say, "I would like to educate myself more about my body, can we go over the results and view the images together?"

Nurses can only do so much because the doctor makes the final call in the treatment of the patient. Nurses can offer different solutions and pose questions to doctors, but many doctors ignore the nurses' requests, thinking themselves to be the smarter and more qualified of the pair.

Another story that illustrates this point…. A patient who was having multiple complications came in for treatment of a UTI and kidney infection. Although it was apparent that her abdominal pain was from the kidney infection/UTI she had, the doctor ordered an EGD to examine her esophagus, stomach, and duodenum. She was not vomiting blood or having gastric issues, so there was really no logical reason to perform this test. Her diabetes and respiratory complications made her a high-risk case which was even more reason not to perform the EGD unless necessary. To top it off, she was also taking Eliquis, a hardcore blood thinner meant to prevent life-threatening blood clots like deep vein thrombosis and pulmonary embolisms. The medication itself comes with a warning that no procedure should be performed while the patient is taking Eliquis due to an elevated risk of the patient bleeding. Patients should be off this medication for 3-5 days and at a minimum of 24 hours before having any procedure done unless it is urgent. We nurses saw that the doctor intended to perform the EGD the next day without waiting for the patient to get off the blood thinner and get her blood clotting abilities back. We called our management and told them that it was contraindicated to do this procedure while the patient was on Eliquis. The management agreed this wasn't an urgent procedure but told us that if the anesthesiologist was on board, the procedure would happen. At this point, I called the doctor himself and told him he should reschedule the EGD since the patient was still taking Eliquis and the response I got was sickening.

"I don't care. Nobody's going to tell me how to do *my* job!" was his ego-centric reply.

The doctor proceeded to do the EGD and found nothing, but as you can see, this doctor did not have the patient's safety in mind. I tell you these things so you can understand what goes on behind the scenes. There are a lot of things the patient and their family don't see, hear, or understand.

One last story for this section. I was the ER nurse for a 2-year-old child with pneumonia. The doctor that was treating her decided that she was okay to be discharged home after her diagnosis and treatment. I was very adamant that she wasn't ready to go home and that she should be admitted for I.V. antibiotics and monitoring. Her oxygen level was only 92% and she was using accessory muscles to breathe.

The mother was getting quite upset over the blatant disregard for her daughter's care and stated herself that her child was still extremely uncomfortable, as she was. When I approached the doctor about this, he shooed me away and said, "Discharge her". I went to the mother and said, "I tried to get her admitted. But the doc thinks she will be fine at home." This distressed the mother greatly and I understood why... because I did not want to discharge her home either. The mother decided to refuse to take her home, and the doctor decided to pretty much ignore her. Eventually, I went to the physician's assistant that had witnessed all the encounters and she agreed with my assessment of the child. I asked her to please go speak with the doctor about this because I am NOT signing my name on those discharge orders. Luckily, she did, and we got the child's pediatrician involved with the case. Her pediatrician came in, assessed her, and was in agreement with the mother and me.

It was a good thing I fought for this child because she ended up in the hospital for a week and a half! When I made a report regarding the incident I was told, "Well, the doc is going through some rough times right now." I said, "And this gives him the right to treat the patient like that, and to disregard me?" After this incident, I was on the doctor's shit list for reporting the incident and protecting the patient and the hospital from liability. Instead of the doctor coming to me and thanking me for having his back (saving his ASS!), I was his enemy.

Things didn't go well for me at that hospital after this incident. This is what I got for being a patient's advocate! The moral of the story: When the shit hits the fan it rolls downhill and guess who's at the bottom... your nurse! This is a big reason nurses tend to keep their mouths shut and another reason YOU need to be your own advocate!

Okay, I know I told you only one more story... but the more I work at various places, the more stories I hear as I draft this book. This is important, especially important. Dr. Accarelli was a doc I used to work with, and he was having symptoms of a stroke. He went to the closest emergency department (not the one he worked at), knew he was having a stroke, and requested T-Pase (clot buster). The Neurologist that was on call refused to give it to him because she did not think he was having a stroke. He and his family knew the risks of the drug and were willing to take them as he was getting worse by the hour, but the doc still refused. By 4 am he was hemiplegic (paralyzed on one side of his body). The staff tried multiple times to get the doctor to come back in and evaluate him, but they wouldn't. By the time the family got one of his co-workers to come in, it was too late to give the T-Pase. This doctor was negligent! Apparently, this wasn't the only time this doc had done something negligent. There had been many complaints from other doctors, nurses, and family members, yet they are still working. You wonder why…

So, when docs do something that gets reported, it undergoes a "peer review". In this review, the doc's name is known, and they go over what occurred and if any discipline or new standards need to be recommended. Think about this, why would any peer of a doctor recommend discipline, when they know they could be reviewed and recommended for discipline themselves? If you are thinking, "THEY WOULDN'T!" you are correct. We need an independent anonymous counsel that DOES NOT know the doctors to review cases and make recommendations. These should be people that aren't working as MDs with the public, so they aren't swayed in their decision-making process. This would help a TON and could even be considered evidence-based practice research to help prevent more errors and create new standard operating procedures.

Unfortunately, the only recourse we have is to sue the hospital and/or the doctor for the incident. Most of us don't have that kind of money or time, and you will likely lose anyways because you are fighting an empire!

This doctor did sue for this incident. Unfortunately,

some "professionals" lied on the stand, and even though there was documentation proving his side and witnesses (the charge nurse and other nurses) that corroborated his story, he lost. It helps to have the judge under your thumb… When he complained about the judge's bias and won an appeal, he could not afford another $450,000 dollars to appeal the case. The hospital knew this to be the case. So, they used their enormous pocketbook to continue the fight knowing he wouldn't have the money to appeal.

Do you wonder why the witnesses lied on the stand? Because they were worried about retaliation and their jobs. Blacklisting is extremely common in medicine even though it is illegal. I hear more and more about blacklisting, and unfortunately, it's the docs that are trying to do the right thing that get blacklisted. You would not believe the number of doctors and upper echelon within the hospital management system that want to tell me their stories, anonymously of course. They don't tell me to stop writing my book. They say, "Please write the book, people need to know!" It happens to nurses too! We have a legal system NOT a justice system. Justice is bleeding from behind her blindfold. **It's time to demand change!**

I hope that reading these few stories (out of hundreds that I have) has made you more aware of how doctors make mistakes and become overloaded and careless with their patients as they get jaded, frustrated, and beaten down throughout their careers. For this reason, you really need to be the squeaky wheel that gets the doctor's grease.

Don't accept everything the doctor says or does. Demand a specialist, demand diagnostics, and demand to see your results. Becoming an active participant in your healthcare will increase your chances of getting out alive. Remember what a doctor recently told me: "You want to live? Stay out of the hospital."

As we will talk about in part 2, it is in your best interest to keep a health advocate on speed dial so they can help you navigate your way through treatment. They can help fight for your rights, decipher your test results, advise you regarding life threatening procedures, and demand care from your doctor when they are being nonchalant about your treatment. You don't have to do it alone.

PART

2

Self Advocacy and Finding a Trusted Health Advocate

Enough scary stories, we need some solutions already. Now you have a solid grasp on the problems of America's healthcare system and why it's important to look out for yourself. The second half of this book is devoted to educating you on how to be the best self-advocate you can be. You've got to understand your rights and how to stand up for yourself and get the care you deserve. Nobody wants a doctor that cares about them less than 100% or one that is constantly making mistakes. But it does happen, and as you've seen in the stories I've shared, it's important to be on the lookout.

Having a family member who works in the medical field can be helpful when trying to understand what's going on. But not everyone is lucky enough to have a family member in the medical field. If this is the case, ask a friend who is and is willing to come fight for your rights and care every step of the way. Even if you do not know anyone who is a medical professional, having someone there with you can help guide the exam and ask questions when you're overwhelmed. Having an advocate will help you get the care you deserve. Even when they are not medical professionals, having two brains in the room will really help. Bring along a good friend or family member.

Being your own health advocate and standing up for your rights as the patient takes courage, questions, and relentless documentation. It also takes someone who is willing to put in the work to research and understand their situation. Many people like to be spoon fed information by their doctor. However, educating yourself about your situation will give you a bigger picture and help you understand it in a way that the doctor probably can't explain to you in 15 minutes or less. Empowering yourself through education will help you to feel more in control throughout the process. You NEED to take responsibility for yourself, I can't stress this enough!

There is no shame in asking for help, medicine is complicated. I know the pitfalls of the medical system and how to avoid them. I know terminology that would take the layperson years to learn. I understand which medications treat which conditions. I have helped treat patients with just about every health condition imaginable during my

16 years in the medical field. How much more confident would you feel if you had someone like that on speed dial? Whoever it is, find someone early. You never know what can happen, trust me.

In Part 2, I will teach you how to become more involved in your own healthcare and how to be proactive while asking the right questions and fighting for your rights. I'll teach you how to communicate with your doctor, I'll discuss alternatives to pharmaceuticals, where to look for legitimate health information, how to stay out of the hospital, and how to develop a medical journal. I don't have all the answers. However, I can guide you in the right direction and empower you with knowledge for better respect and treatment from your healthcare team.

CHAPTER 6

SELF DIAGNOSIS AND INVESTIGATIVE RESEARCH

I find it funny how much doctors hate the power that technology has given patients. They complain about how annoying it is that everyone thinks they can diagnose themselves through Web MD.

Personally, I love it. I love that there is so much information out there educating people about how their body works, how a disease works, and what could be going wrong with their health. It empowers people. It clues people into their own health. Before, only doctors had the information that people needed. This created a huge power imbalance, with the layperson clueless and helpless, meanwhile, some doctors get drunk on their own wine because they are the only ones with the knowledge and the answers to help.

If doctors see that you know your stuff and you are

not coming to them clueless, they will take you more seriously and think more carefully about their treatment approach, recognizing your knowledge is a tool to hold them accountable. Nowadays, however, most people will google their condition even before making a doctor's appointment. I think this can lighten the load on hospitals and doctors because patients can determine the severity of their condition before panicking and going to the hospital. Conversely, it could also save lives because a patient could learn their persistent annoying symptoms could be part of a more serious condition.

It's important when doing your own research to remember that many symptoms are the same for various conditions. For example, googling "cause of abdominal pain" will reveal that you could be having indigestion, food allergies, a virus, or cancer of the stomach. These conditions vary greatly in their severity so don't let yourself panic. Remember, just because you are researching doesn't mean you have the answer. Oftentimes, only an MRI or other diagnostic test can confirm the cause of discomfort.

Many people DO freak themselves out because most thorough medical articles will list all the probable causes of a symptom, from the least severe to the most severe. It's important to take everything you read with a grain of salt. You have a unique body and have a unique situation going on. Resist the brain's temptation to jump to the worst-case scenario right away.

Learning about what you can do immediately to improve your condition will likely help you feel more empowered. For example, if you have been getting headaches everyday and you google this, you will find that your headache could be the result of chronic dehydration. Our brains are 70-80% water so being dehydrated directly impacts the brain's feeling and function. Instead of rushing to the doctor wondering if you have a brain tumor, start drinking water. If dehydration is the cause of the headache, it will go away within a day or two given you keep your water levels up. Not only did you fix your own health problem (helping you regain a sense of power in your own life), you also just built a healthy habit that will prevent other conditions. All because of the information sharing going on across the internet.

Another benefit of educating yourself about your condition is being taken more seriously by your doctors and nurses. Learning anatomy and medical terminology will make you sound so much smarter in the doctor's office or hospital and could get you better care. <u>KNOWLEDGE IS POWER.</u>

With that being said, it's important to do your research on reputable sites that have articles written by doctors, nurses, and scientists, NOT snake oil salesmen. Many blogs just regurgitate information from other sites, not always accurately at that. Consider the source of the article you are reading. Does the writer have some medical background that makes them a credible source? Or do they have some bonehead degree, thinking of themselves as a know it all? COVID exposed this all too well. Please make sure you're getting your information from reputable sources.

A few websites I recommend using for your research are:

WebMD

This website provides accurate, scientific, up to date health information and is run by doctors. Every article is reviewed by at least one board certified physician. Content created by Web MD is free from advertiser influences and other outside sources that are not medical professionals. The editorial team is kept separate from the advertising team so as not to skew information based on special interests. This is what has made this site such a trusted source of information.

Instead of waiting to ask your doctor questions, you can get information from several doctors who have experience in the field. The site does come with this warning, however: "Never disregard professional medical advice or delay in seeking it because of something you have read on the WebMD Site!"

WebMD has a wide variety of articles addressing a plethora of health conditions. Almost any condition you will experience has a corollary article on this site. The site also features a symptom checker, a list of the best hospitals and doctors, information on prescription drugs and interactions between them, along with articles on prevention and healthy living. This site has a plethora of information, and I would strongly encourage you to use it for your research.

Mayo Clinic

Mayo Clinic is another reputable site for medical research. The site has articles on hundreds of diseases and conditions. With over 70 board certified physicians on the editorial team, you know you are getting the most up to date accurate medical information you can get.

The site also has a symptom checker, information on drugs and supplements, along with articles about tests and procedures. Mayo Clinic's "Health Information" tab also offers recommended books for healthy living, and they really emphasize a healthy lifestyle as a key to prevention and disease management. As with WebMD, they stress the importance of seeing your doctor to get the individual care you need instead of relying on articles to definitively diagnose your condition.

The Mayo Clinic itself has a reputation for helping those that other doctors and hospitals could not. The Clinic has been ranked the top hospital nationwide for many years. Mayo Clinic physicians are the best in their fields and receive salary pay so they never need to make decisions about patient care based on monetary issues. The bedrock of the Clinic's philosophy is "patient-first".

With this commitment to the best care possible, they have been able to treat a variety of complex health conditions with high rates of success.

If you are experiencing a complicated medical issue that no one can seem to help you with, you may consider reaching out to Mayo Clinic to set up an appointment with one of their trusted and experienced physicians. If you are still in the research phase, you can count on accurate information from this site.

National Institute of Health

Part of the US Department of Health and Human Services, The National Institutes of Health is the world's largest medical library. There is a wealth of information and research on this site. If you love sinking your teeth into research papers, this medical research agency is your happy place. PubMed, part of the NIH library, is the most trusted resource for biomedical and life sciences literature on the internet.

MedlinePlus

MedlinePlus is a government run website that is part of the National Library of Medicine. In addition to their information on drugs, supplements, diseases, and procedures, they also have information about genetics. This includes information on genetic conditions, how genes are linked to health, gene therapy, and more. Enjoy the benefits of a massive database.

Testing.com

Everything you need to know about lab tests can be found on testing.com. Their tagline sums up their mission: "Understand your tests. Empower your health." Understand how lab tests work and how to interpret them. Any type of testing that gets sent to the lab will be explained on this site. Some examples are:

- Anemia
- Fertility
- STDs
- CBC (complete blood count)
- Urinalysis
- Pneumonia
- Sleep Apnea
- Thyroid Function
- Glucose
- Iron
- And many more

This site also has home testing kits available for allergies, strep throat, STD's, Lyme disease, cholesterol, herpes, COVID-19, and many others.

You can also look into college textbooks from nursing school. These books are unbiased, have an entire range of information on healthcare, and are a fantastic source.

The next section is going to discuss how to create a medical journal and maintain it. As we get older, we tend to forget about past conditions or problems we have had. This is an essential source of information for you and your doctor throughout your whole life. These are the things as an ER nurse I found could have made the difference between life and death for some patients. So, I really recommend that you create one.

The Medical Journal

Everyone should have a medical journal. In that journal is all your medical history. I recommend that you get all your medical records from all your doctors and put them in your journal. You may have to streamline them to make the journal manageable. Our system is severely lacking in keeping your records. That way if you ever end up seeing another doctor, you don't have to go through the long painful process of getting your records which delays your care and can end up with disastrous results.

It should also have your advanced directive (your wishes if something really bad happens to you) in it. If you're completely incapacitated, someone should be able to give this journal to an emergency room doctor and they should be able to treat you fully and completely with a greater chance of survival. All this information should be in the front of the journal or on a thumb drive. The rest of the journal should be pages for you to document your daily health issues or conditions when they occur. That template I gave to you in this book for you to fill out for your purse or wallet should be the first page. It's a quick emergency reference for anyone needing it. Plus, being in two places has a higher likelihood of being seen.

When you first start experiencing symptoms of any health problem, I recommend that you start writing things down right away in your medical journal.

- When did the symptoms start, date/time?
- Does it come and go or is it persistent?
- If it does come and go, how long does it last?
- If you have pain, is it sharp, dull, burning, or aching? Is it localized or does it radiate/travel?
- How bad is the pain? Scale 1-10, ***BE HONEST!*** 10 is your arm got cut off! This makes a big difference in diagnosis!!! Faking your pain to get drugs DOES NOT help you or the community, it makes your nurses and doctors jaded!!!
- Does activity make it worse? If so, what kind of activity squatting, lifting, running, sitting, etc?
- Does it hurt when you palpate (push) on it or not?
- Does it happen after you eat? Is food involved?
- Is there anything that makes it feel better?
- Does it swell up, if so, what causes it to swell?

Keeping a medical journal is a way for you to keep a record of your condition. When you eventually get to meet with a doctor, you will save so much time and help your doctor out tremendously by bringing your medical journal which has all sorts of valuable information for them. To give your doc even more information about yourself, write down the following:

- Your dietary habits, including anything new that has been added or anything you stopped eating. Also, write down how much water you intake every day.
- Which supplements you are taking and how long you've been taking them.
- Which medications you are on (including dosage) and how long you've been taking them for, including any side effects they have on you. Include which doctor prescribed them to you.
- Anything emotional or traumatic that has happened in your life recently and in the past.

As you do your research, write down in your medical journal anything you find that stands out to you as a possible diagnosis. Of course, you won't always be able to accurately diagnose yourself, but if you show your doctor you have looked into your condition, they will know you are looking for solutions too. You might even give them an idea or two.

Also, write down the medical terminology regarding your condition. If you come to your doctor already speaking their language, they will take you a lot more seriously. Coming to them not just as another clueless patient, but as someone who has done some research to get to the bottom of the problem will earn you a lot more respect from the medical staff. It will also help expedite the process significantly.

Think about it, doctors have so many patients that they have a limited window of time for you. If you can come into your appointment organized with your medical journal and list of questions, you will save the doctor time and help them find the underlying cause of your problem faster (instead of multiple visits costing you money, frustration, and anxiety). Trust me, your doctor will be overly impressed, and you will likely have a better outcome from your visit.

CHAPTER 7

THE ONLY STUPID QUESTION IS THE ONE YOU DON'T ASK

Is my anesthesiologist/attending doctor (doctor taking care of you in the hospital) covered under my insurance?

Can I see my test results with my own eyes?

Can I have a copy of my visit including the doctor's notes, right now, before I leave, not later?

These are all questions that you have every right to ask and should ask if you want the best health outcomes possible. If something happens to you and you don't have access to your local doctors and must wait for your records to be mailed or faxed, it could be too late and you may end up dead. Keep ALL your records of all your important visits, MRI's, CT scans, X-rays, etc. with you in a file or on a thumb drive.

QUESTIONS ARE CRUCIAL.
QUESTIONS SAVE LIVES.

Before your doctor's visit, write down all of the questions you have. Take some time to make a thorough list of anything you don't understand and need to be educated about. A doctor that cares will have no problem answering any medical question you ask them. Most good doctors actually like educating their patients and are impressed when you ask questions that show you truly want to understand your condition.

Bring a piece of paper with all of your questions written down so you don't forget any of them in the daze of the doctor. Also, do not let them talk over you. Make sure they know that they are there to help you, not just to talk at you. Any doctor who does not like questions or tries to rush you out the door is a red flag. Consider switching doctors if this is the case.

Record your office visits with your voice memo app on your phone. This way you have a record and a reference for yourself regarding what the doctor's answers were. Get the doctor's consent before recording, telling the doctor the purpose is to remember what they told you and what you two discussed. Any doctor that has a problem with being recorded is also a huge red flag.

This serves a few purposes. First, you will indeed have a reference to go back to, should you forget what the doctor told you. Secondly, it gives you a record of how your case was treated. So, in the event that the doctor is negligent and denies you the tests you need, you have it all on record. It may also help with any appeals you may need to make in the case of denied care by the health insurance companies. In the next chapter, I'll give you an example of a situation that happened to my mom. Had she recorded her office visits, the doctor would have been held accountable for his blatant lack of care.

There are questions that you may not think to ask, and this is where having a trusted health advocate with you can come in handy. For instance, many people don't know that while in the hospital, their primary doctor may be covered under their insurance, but the attending doctor may not be. Most hospitals won't tell you this and you'll end up getting a huge bill from your attending doctor when you get home. How would you know to ask for an attending doctor that is covered by your insurance unless you knew this crucial piece of information?

"We are far from achieving patient-centered care," claim the authors of a study published in the Journal of General Internal Medicine regarding how much time patients get to speak during their appointment. They found that only 36% of patients are given a chance to talk about why they came in for their visit. Even more shocking, only 20% of patients seeking specialty care were asked what was wrong.

Without balanced patient-doctor communication, patients are often left out of the decision making process.

According to this study, patients only spoke for an average of 11 seconds before doctors interrupted them. Without interruption, patients will speak for about 30-90 seconds about their condition. But due to doctors being so busy and burnt out from dealing with so many patients, they often fail to listen as they should.

Physicians from Harvard have some good advice to increase your chances of being heard:

- Always come to your appointment early
- Have your list of questions in hand
- Bring a health advocate to ensure you are communicating properly and being heard by the doctor
- Disclose any and all information you can, even mentioning the minor symptoms you are having

When formulating a list of questions, they will obviously be specific to your situation. However, there are definitely some basics to cover when it comes to questions. Here are a few ideas:

What could my symptoms indicate?

How can we find out what is going on with me? Do I need blood work and/or diagnostic tests?

Are there symptoms to keep an eye out for?

What can I expect from this test or treatment? Are there any risks involved? What are they?

What are my treatment options for this condition? What is the success rate of these treatments? Are there experimental treatment options? If so, how do I get involved?

Why am I being prescribed this medication? Are there any natural or alternative solutions I can try first or in combination?

What are the side effects of this medication? Is there anything I need to avoid while taking it such as alcohol, supplements, certain foods, etc.? Are there negative long-term effects of being on this medication? REMEMBER TO ASK YOUR PHARMACIST THESE QUESTIONS TOO!

Is there a cheaper version of this medication, perhaps a generic version?

What information did you use to come up with my diagnosis? Are there any other possible reasons for my symptoms?

When will I receive my test results? Will you call me, or should I call you?

Is this covered by my insurance? (Your doc may not know this, ask the front desk to confirm.)

How will my life change due to my condition? What is the progression of this disease and what can I expect in the future?

Are there potential complications from this procedure? What are they? What does this medical term mean?

Also, it's important to ask for a copy of your medical records and the doctor's notes. Some systems such as Kaiser will post your medical history, test results, and doctor's notes online for you to view at your convenience.

If this is not the case for you, I would strongly encourage you to get a copy of your medical record, including doctor's notes, after each visit.

Part of your HIPPA rights entitle you to ask for a copy of any and all medical records the doctor has, including test results and all of the doctor's notes.

Concise record keeping will protect you in the future if the doctor is being negligent or is having difficulty diagnosing you. You will see in the following chapter that had my mom requested her medical records, she could have pressed legal charges against the doctor that caused her a huge amount of unnecessary pain and suffering.

What questions to ask when scheduled for surgery

In the last two years I have been working in several different ASC's (ambulatory surgical centers). I have come to the conclusion that there's a ton of them out there, and many of them are purely unsafe. I commonly work in understaffed conditions in facilities that barely have an established crash cart (the cart we wheel over when you're crashing that has all the lifesaving medications and equipment in it). Some, I had considerable concerns about how sanitary they were. Many had minimal supplies and were running with a skeleton crew, where the pre-op nurse was the recovery nurse, with only one vital sign being monitored.

I worked with a doctor that did an 8-hour tummy tuck and breast reduction procedure. I was the Pre-op, PACU (recovery), and OR nurse. It was done in an office-like setting that he had set up like an OR. I am sure it was done legitimately. But I wouldn't consider it safe. There was only one patient for the day, so I wasn't upset that I was doing all the stations. However, it was kind of a hodgepodge set up if you know what I mean. One monitor for multiple beds, etc. He actually had another patient visit while he was doing the surgery. He scrubbed out, did a minor procedure on the other patient with my help and then scrubbed back in for the 8-hour surgery. Granted, the anesthesiologist was with the surgical patient. But I didn't consider that sanitary or safe. After the 8-hour surgery was completed, the anesthesiologist left pretty much right away and left me with the doctor. This made me quite upset and the doctor had a dinner plan that he insisted on making in 30 minutes. The patient was not coming out of surgery well and was experiencing significant nausea and vomiting. I requested Zofran (anti-nausea medication) and administered it with the doctor's order. He insisted on discharging the patient in that condition, after an 8-hour surgery and only a 30-minute recovery. Normally, we would hold that patient for at least 1 hour. I told him she's not ready to be discharged. But he didn't care and wheeled her out to the car. I told the patient to go to the emergency department for treatment and evaluation because I had considerable concerns about her condition. Needless to say, I reported him to my registry company and refused to go back.

These surgery centers are money makers. Quite a few places have popped up because of this and they are puppy mills. They try to get as many patients in and out as fast as possible, you are a dollar bill to them. These centers do have to get certified. However, many get by with just the minimum needed for certification and then after they pass certification standards, they loosen up on safety requirements until it's time to pass again. There are many places I refuse to work because I worry about my license and the safety of the patients at these locations.

What this means to you is that you must do your research when prepping for a procedure.

- Ask about the location of the procedure
- Request a tour of the facility
- Inquire about who your anesthesiologist will be
- Ask when their last health inspection was, and did they pass the first time
- How many nurses will they have and what will the nurse-to-patient ratio be
- What are their emergency protocols and is the crash cart stocked appropriately
- How long will your stay be for recovery
- What is their infection rate

- Are the staff all per diem registry or actual staff members
- How long has the surgery center been open

When you do your walk-through of the facility, pay attention to cleanliness. Do the walls look clean, is the paint peeling, is there mold or blood? How many beds do they have, and does each one have a monitor? What do the monitors look like? Are they in working condition and clean? Is there oxygen available at each station along with a bedside table with its own blood pressure cuff, etc. Are the floors clean, is there a wheelchair available and is it clean? Are there curtains to separate you from other patients, and what do the beds look like? Inspect for blood on the railings and the mattress. What is the overall impression of the facility? It should look tidy, organized, and exceptionally clean.

These are all especially important questions when it comes to your safety as a patient. I would reconsider any procedure where they are reluctant to let you tour the facility. In my experience, the safest facilities are the ones associated with a hospital system or a large corporation. Don't be afraid to ask these tough questions, it's your life on the line. If your gut is telling you, *this place makes my skin crawl*, then it's probably correct. Don't take the chance.

CHAPTER 8

WHEN TO DEMAND A DIAGNOSTIC TEST

My mom went to the dermatologist because she was concerned about a growth on the inside of her nose. She knew something wasn't right because the growth felt abnormal, and it had intermittent bleeding. She went to the dermatologist and told him she thought it should get looked at, and maybe biopsied, and that she was very concerned it was cancer. He said it didn't look like anything serious and sent her away.

1 month later, my mom went back to her dermatologist because the growth was bleeding a lot and was sore. "I really think I need a biopsy," said my mom, concerned. He finally agreed to biopsy it.

And what do you know? The lab results showed the growth to be an aggressive Morpheaform basal cell carcinoma. Instead of sending my mom to the hospital to get the proper surgery to remove the cancer the right way, he sent her to get a MOHs surgery in an office. A MOHs surgery is a procedure where doctors cut the cancer off layer by layer, testing the layers as they go. The idea is to cut out all the edges of the cancer while leaving the healthy tissue intact.

Since my mom's dermatologist had waited so long to do the biopsy, the cancer had spread quite a bit. During the MOHs surgery, the doctors excised more and more tissue away. Instead of stopping and saying, "we need to finish this in an operating room", they continued to inject lidocaine over and over (which in itself is extremely dangerous and can cause heart arrhythmias) until _half of my mom's nose was missing, with NO PAIN MEDICATION!_ Lidocaine only lasts so long. My mom was completely traumatized, watching half her nose disappear and having terrible pain, so I flew to Colorado to be with her and to advocate for her care.

By the time I got to my mom, she was starting to run a fever. She is allergic to almost all antibiotics, so if she got an infection, it could kill her. She desperately needed surgery to fix her nose and cover up the hole that was now in her face. Her insurance company was trying to weasel their way out of covering her surgery, saying it was cosmetic. My step dad tried twice and got nowhere. So, I got on the phone with them right away:

"I'm going to own you! If my mom gets an infection and she dies, _I will own your company. WHO THE HELL ARE YOU TO TELL ME THIS IS COSMETIC!!!!_

SHE DOESN'T EVEN HAVE A NOSE ANYMORE!!! So, this is how this is going to go, **YOU ARE GOING TO DO THIS!** You are going to call the doctor, call the hospital, get in touch with *WHOMEVER* you need to get in touch with to make this surgery happen **TODAY!**" The insurance company was actually going to try to weasel their way out of providing a crucial surgery. Mind you, they had denied facial laser surgery the year before for multiple pre-cancers on her face! Had she gotten that done, who knows, this may have never happened. I made sure to mention this in our conversation, for the record.

Anyway, they knew I meant business and sure enough, the surgery happened that night. By the time my mom went into surgery, she was already starting to get an infection and was running a fever of 102.0 degrees. During the surgery, the doctor cut a flap of skin and an artery from her forehead and did a living graft to give her a nose again. It was a 7-hour surgery!

My mom, in addition to being incredibly traumatized and in horrible pain, had to live with a living graft on her face *for a whole month*. Kids and adults alike would stare at her, making her feel like a complete monster! I had to take a month off of work to help manage the living graft to make sure it would take; she wasn't out of the woods yet. She still needed a second surgery to trim the living graft after the tissue healed into the other tissues on her nose. Imagine what that would feel like! All because the doctor wouldn't do a biopsy in the first place!

When we went back to her dermatologist for a follow up after the second surgery, he treated her like absolute garbage. Instead of being apologetic that he didn't take a biopsy sooner, causing tremendous pain and suffering, he was a complete asshole. He even had another doctor in the room to "witness" the appointment. When we left the office, we were both baffled.

"What the hell was that all about?" I asked my mom.

"I don't know," she responded, "but he's a total asshole."

The reason was he was a complete and utter jerk-face... He knew that he screwed up. He knew he should have ordered the biopsy the first time my mom came in with a sore in her nose. She already had multiple cancers taken off her face and her back (at least 10) which would have given any good doctor a reason to biopsy the sore right away.

Everybody makes mistakes, but the utter disrespect and meanness of the doctor after causing so much pain and suffering made us get a lawyer. However, we didn't get very far in taking legal action against this doctor before we found out that he had falsified my mother's medical records. In her file, the doctor wrote that he had offered to take a biopsy of my mother's sore, and my mother refused. He knew she had every right to sue his pants off, so he blatantly broke the law and altered the medical records, changing the history of what really happened. No lawyer would take the case. They said, "It's your word against his, I am sorry."

Why would my mother make her own appointment to go into the dermatologist and then refuse a biopsy?

On top of that, the process wasn't completely done yet. She still needed a third surgery to complete the septum and shape the nose for better breathing. WE WERE NOT GOING TO GO BACK TO HIM! So, my mom tried multiple different doctors and couldn't find one that would finish the procedure, due to the fact that the records showed she refused care at one point... Which was complete BULLSHIT! SHE HAD BEEN BLACKLISTED!!! All because of one doctor's ignorance and falsification of records to protect his own ass!

This story isn't over yet, adding insult to injury! When the medical bills started pouring in, the insurance company wanted to deny paying them, claiming that my mother caused her own problem by denying the biopsy! They actually told her that maybe she needs social services to help her take care of herself!!! WTF!?! We eventually got the insurance company to pay, that was a major needless battle! You don't want to be this victim. So, do your due diligence!

I had my own experience with being sent away when I really should have had a biopsy taken.

I had found a growth on the back of my head that started to bleed. I also had this yellowish foul-smelling discharge from the same area—a warning sign!

"This doesn't look good to me. This might be something to be concerned about," I said adamantly to my dermatologist. (Mind you, I have a family history of skin cancer and have had it before myself.)

"It's fine, nothing to be worried about," was her unprofessional, irresponsible response. I pushed for a biopsy. I figured, why take a chance? Who does it hurt except me? But she actually told me, "I don't have time to do a biopsy today and it looks fine to me." *YOU DON'T HAVE THE TIME!?! Why the Hell am I here then?* was my thought. I should have said it!

A month later it was bleeding again. I didn't want to go to her, but it was months before I could get an appointment to see someone else, so I went in, determined to get it biopsied. Sure enough, it was squamous cell cancer... the kind of cancer that can metastasize.

Well, jeez, I could have *told* you that. In fact, I *did* tell you that! But you didn't want to biopsy it. Now I have a large scar on the back of my head after getting a huge chunk of tissue removed.

These painful personal experiences have taught me to trust my gut and demand a biopsy when I think I need one. If your gut is telling you something, your body is telling you something. **TRUST YOUR GUT!** Trust yourself more than what the doctors are telling you. Don't let any doctor or nurse talk you out of what your intuition is telling you. It's not worth your life or the suffering that will come as a result of their negligence.

The body has its own wisdom and will communicate to you if only you will listen. I have seen too many people end up in health crises or 6 feet under because they trusted the doctor more than they trusted themselves. Nobody knows your body better than you. You are the master and commander, and when your ship needs repair, you know it. I can't tell you how many times I hear patients tell me, "I wish I would've listened to my gut."

If they keep trying to brush off your concerns, always get a second opinion. Find someone who will do the biopsy and do it fast. Some cancers are fast growing and it's good to find out what it is as soon as possible and get it out.

If you have a bad feeling about it, trust it. Tell your doctor you want a biopsy or whatever test it is to rule out a disease as soon as possible. Especially mention if you have a family history or personal history of cancer or other disease processes. And of course, get it all on record.

Voice record all of your doctor visits.

Everybody has a voice memo app on their phone, right? How hard is it to pull out your cell phone and tell the doctor you are going to record the appointment so you can remember what he/she told you? It's totally valid to want to remember the doctor's terminology and instructions, so they should have no problem with it. If they do, you should be very wary and possibly find another doctor.

Along with holding them accountable for what they say, you are also encouraging them to be on their best behavior, giving you the best treatment possible. :)

And truly, using it for your own purposes is valid. How many times have you walked out of the doctor's office and immediately asked yourself, "What did they say that condition was called? What's the medication they are giving me? What was it they wanted me to do?" It's good record keeping, just like your medical journal. If you don't record it, at least write it down.

If my mom had recorded her doctor refusing to biopsy, she would have had a solid case against him. But when it's the patient's word versus the doctor's word, guess who wins most of the time? You got it, the doctor.

Many times, it's the insurance companies that are the ones who deny coverage of diagnostic tests. If your doctor knows your insurance will not cover a certain test, they may opt to give you a band-aid in the form of prescription medication. In this way, they can help you feel better and ease your discomfort, while offering a solution that your insurance will actually pay for. This is how the opioid crisis came about. Instead of getting to the bottom of people's pain through expensive diagnostics, doctors instead put a band-aid on it with opioids, causing lifelong addictions and countless overdoses.

Even when doctors want to do the right thing, often insurance companies get in the way of the proper care being distributed, causing frustration for doctors and patients alike. Remember, in many other countries, insurance companies cannot legally deny any medical claims. But in our for-profit healthcare system, insurance companies pick and choose what to pay for based on their determination of necessity.

Do doctors work for insurance companies and advise them to accept or deny certain claims? *Yes, and they get paid big bonuses for limiting insurance companies' losses!* They get a salary, work from home, get good benefits, retirement… this is another story entirely! Does this sound beneficial to you?

Why do insurance companies get to accept or deny claims based on what they think is necessary? They should leave what is necessary to a doctor and their patient and cover the expenses that are needed. This is how it should be, anyway. Remember this is how it is done in most other countries.

What we actually have with health insurance is a group of pencil pushers trying to save their company as much money as possible to increase their profit margins while having absolutely no clue nor concern about what the patient actually needs.

Getting a voice recording of your visits can help you with a medical claim. If you told the doctor your symptoms and they recommended something, shouldn't your medical insurance cover it? You are holding everybody liable—the doctors, the administrators, and the insurance companies.

There are a lot of technicalities with insurance companies, and you can't always know what they will cover and when. Being your own health advocate means keeping records and collecting evidence as a lawyer would. Have things put in writing and take recordings. Document what happens with all of the doctors and nurses taking care of you.

Of course, always get consent before getting a voice recording. A health care professional refusing to be recorded is a sign they don't want their actions and words documented which should set off alarm bells in your head.

So, when should you demand a diagnostic test? And which kind?

Let's start with skin cancer because this is the easiest thing to visually examine. Doctors recommend checking the skin on your whole body at least once per month. Use a full- length mirror and a second handheld mirror to view the back of your body. If you have a partner or family member who you are comfortable with, they can help you check the areas you cannot see, like your scalp and back.

For a self-exam, complete the following steps:

> **Step 1**: Standing in front of a mirror, check your face, ears, neck, chest, and belly. Women may need to lift their breast tissue to check underneath.

> **Step 2**: Next, check your armpits, your entire arms, both sides of your hands, between the fingers, and even underneath the fingernails as cancerous growths can form here too.

Step 3: Sitting down, examine the front of your legs, top of the feet, in between toes, and underneath the toenails.

Step 4: Take your handheld mirror and use it to examine the bottoms of your feet and the backs of your calves and thighs.

Step 5: Standing back up, check the buttocks, genital area, your entire back, neck, and behind the ears.

Step 6: Use a comb or hair dryer to examine the entirety of your scalp.

Consider making it a habit to do this skin check after you get out of the shower and before you get dressed. If this is the first time you have done a skin check, take the time to closely examine every part of your body and take note of all the moles, freckles, and other skin spots you have. This way, when you do your next self-exam, you can see if anything has changed in size, shape, color, or consistency.

- **A:** area (size)
- **B:** borders (irregular shape)
- **C:** color (very dark, or changes color)

Make a note of anything that looks strange or is painful to the touch in your medical journal. Also, consider taking close up pictures of it as time progresses so you have a record to show the doctor how it has changed.

Familiarize yourself with how skin cancer can look by doing a quick google image search. Cancer.org also has an image gallery of several types of skin cancer. Compare your own skin spots with the pictures you find. Also, keep your eyes out for:

- A growth that is new, is growing, or has changed
- A sore that bleeds and doesn't heal over several weeks
- A mole with irregular borders, an odd shape, or areas of differing colors
- A wart-like growth
- A scaly rough red patch that may bleed or crust over

If you have anything that fits these criteria, or something that just doesn't look right and you don't have a good feeling about, demand a biopsy. If the doctor refuses, ask them why not? Also, ask if you can record him refusing to biopsy you and see if that changes their tune.

As far as internal symptoms are concerned, any persistent pain warrants a deeper look. Remember my patient with stage 4 bone cancer whose doctor refused to do any diagnostic testing on? If the patient had trusted his gut and demanded an X-ray, they could have caught the cancer earlier in its development. But because the doctor wrote it off as a minor issue that wasn't to be concerned about because he was young and the patient didn't know any better but to trust his doctor, he is now in a world of hurt and quite possibly may not even survive at this point. While doctors do have the right to refuse to order diagnostic testing for a patient, you have a few options. You can ask to be referred to a specialist, you can be persistent with the doctor in asking for a test, or you can find a new doctor who will be more receptive to your concerns. Whatever you do, don't give up. You may think, "oh it's really nothing, the doc thinks it's nothing." It is your life, not theirs. You may pay dearly for that nonchalant attitude. TRUST YOUR GUT!

CHAPTER 9

LEARNING HOW TO HOLD YOUR GROUND WITH DOCTORS

I had knee surgery when I was 16 years old. Because of a mistake the surgeon made, I had chronic pain for the next 15 years of my life. I would go to see doctors regularly to tell them about my pain and try to find a solution. They would tell me I was crazy, that it was all in my head, and that I didn't have any pain! After hearing this over and over again, I started putting it on myself, thinking maybe it was all in my head and wondering if something was wrong with me mentally. What was their solution? They just put me on a pain medication called Gabapentin, which was awful trying to get off, the withdrawals were INSANE!! I quit the stuff after I got into an accident. One of the side effects is slowed response times. I realized after the accident that maybe I would have avoided the accident altogether if I didn't feel so slow. A broken nose, concussion, burns on both my arms and my face, and a totaled vehicle pushed me to start searching for a doctor that was willing to help.

I finally found a good doctor who decided to take me seriously. Guess what he discovered? The screw that had been put in my knee 15 years ago was TOO LONG! He proposed a surgical procedure to take it out. Sure enough, during surgery, my doctor discovered that the screw which was too long had been rubbing against the nerve in the back of my leg… for 15 years!

I WAS having legitimate pain; I was in fact not crazy and should never have been treated as such. But being young and naive, and not having any of the knowledge and experience I have now, I let the doctors dismiss the very real pain that I was having. If I had known to stand my ground with my doctors, I would have demanded every diagnostic test I could get until I found the problem. Instead, I let doctors walk all over me, telling me that I wasn't feeling the pain that I was in fact feeling, or that I would just have to live with the pain.

6 months after the screw was taken out of my knee, the pain was completely gone. What a long-awaited relief that was! If doctors had listened to me instead of projecting their ego based assumptions onto me, I could have gotten my problem fixed a heck of a lot sooner! This was a very painful lesson that I really needed to hold my ground with doctors. Trust your body and its messages and don't let the doctors talk you out of your symptoms.

Doctors can be real jerks sometimes. I've experienced this many times working closely with them. Some good doctors become jaded and burnt-out, frustrated by the system. I know some docs that literally left the country to work somewhere else because they were so frustrated. Some are full of themselves and think they can make no mistakes. And some just plain don't care about their patients anymore and are only in it for the money.

Of course, there are a lot of genuinely caring and concerned doctors out there who got into this profession for the right reasons and are great at their jobs. Do your research, ask around, and find the one that is right for you. I've had a few amazing doctors that really cared, and I hung onto them like glue! My ER docs were amazing. I still refer to them when something comes up with my health. ER doctors are a different breed. They actually do watch patients decline in front of their eyes. They get that "gut feeling" as well. Although, they are becoming extremely jaded because of the number of patients they see due to the declining availability of healthcare in this country. **Please, only go to the emergency room for an EMERGENCY!!!**

Anyways, at some point in your life, you will likely have to deal with one of these unpleasant doctors that wants you out of their office as soon as possible. They will find the quickest fix (often a pill), write you a prescription, and send you on your way. The problem with this is often the root cause of the problem is never addressed, only the symptoms.

Many doctors have created opioid addictions in

thousands of patients by prescribing a band-aid instead of getting to the root cause of the pain. The problem with pain medication is that you are silencing your body's very important communication system. Pain is a signal that there is a problem. By blocking pain signals, the actual problem never gets better and often gets worse.

As the body builds a tolerance to these opioids, it starts creating new pain receptors in an effort to get the message to the brain that something is wrong. Over time, people need to start taking more pain medication to get the same relief because there are now double the amount of pain receptors! This explains why it is so hard to get off of these powerful opioids. Now that the patient has double their pain receptors, they have double the amount of pain when not using the opioids! The discomfort is so great when trying to go off pain medications that many people choose to stay on them indefinitely.

Don't settle for a band-aid treatment because your doctor can't find the solution. Find another doctor and do your own research to get to the bottom of your pain. Find natural and holistic ways to treat this pain before using powerful, addictive narcotics.

The main complaint I hear from people is that their doctor just doesn't listen to them. If you are in this situation, make it known to your doctor that you are not feeling heard and that your needs are not being addressed. Carry the attitude with you that the doctor is there to serve you, not the other way around. Your pain is valid. Your symptoms are valid. Your questions are valid. Don't let your doctor or any medical professional silence you or make you feel crazy for stating your symptoms and concerns.

I can tell you this, I would much rather prefer a Nurse Practitioner as my main healthcare provider than a doctor. They are required to have a certain number of years of experience as a bedside nurse before they can even apply to college to be an RNP. Your nurse is the one calling the doctor to let them know that their patient isn't looking good, that something is not right. We have watched patients decline before our very eyes; doctors don't get that. We have developed the "gut" feeling because we are constantly with our patients. The average doctor is lucky to spend 10 minutes at the patient's bedside, not enough time to develop a "gut" feeling. Most RNPs have a great bedside manner because we have developed one as a nurse. We learned how to listen to our patients and take advice from our team without letting our egos get in the way.

When a nurse practitioner walks in the room to treat you, be happy you got one. You will likely enjoy your treatment and care if you give them a chance. When there is an option for a nurse practitioner in the medical group, make that choice, you won't regret it. If you have concerns about experience, a RNP is working under a physician and can refer to them if needed. So, you get the best of both worlds.

It's important to understand that you have a choice in your treatment. You have the right to say "yes" or "no" to any test, treatment, drug, or surgery that your doctor proposes.

After doing your own research, you may find that the risks of a procedure outweigh the benefits and you may try to find another solution outside of surgery. I have known a few people who have been able to prevent carpal tunnel surgery by receiving massage therapy, for example.

Some patients with late-stage diseases or in their old age would rather not put themselves through traumatic treatments like chemo or risky surgeries. Some patients decide they want to live out their days at home, not going in and out of surgery. Every patient has the right to choose what is best for their life.

No conversation about patient rights would be complete without talking about HIPAA rights.

In 1996, the Health Insurance Portability and Accountability Act (HIPAA) became federal law. HIPAA was originally intended to help individuals continue to have health insurance coverage after leaving their jobs. Over time, it was expanded to include laws about patient privacy and rights to medical records.

HIPPA RIGHTS:

Every patient has a right to get a copy of their medical records from:

- Doctors
- Hospitals
- Pharmacies

- Laboratories
- Health Insurance Plans

This includes everything your doctor has ordered including tests, medications, and procedures. It also includes all doctors' notes and test results. You are entitled to get a copy of these records in a timely fashion. Nobody can refuse to give you your records, even if you have not paid your medical bill yet.

You are also entitled to have a copy of your records sent to other people (such as family members and caregivers) along with sending information to a health app to be used for health tracking. While doctors are encouraged to give you a copy of your medical records for free, some charge a small fee and require forms to request a copy.

Doctors are required to inform you if there will be a fee to get a copy of your health records. This fee is required to be minimal, only covering the cost of supplies and postage if you are being mailed a paper copy. They must also get them to you within 30 days of your request.

If you see an error on your medical record, you can submit a correction. Even if the doctor doesn't change it right away, your note will be in your medical record that you want to correct an error on your file. You can also submit a complaint if you think your rights were violated.

Under HIPAA laws, no one is allowed to see your medical record without your consent. Of course, medical staff will have access to it, but if any family member or friend tries to see your file, they will not be able to without your permission.

Hospitals and doctors' offices are required to implement security measures to make sure your information doesn't get into the wrong hands. They must safely guard your medical records through cyber security and physical security. Although many records are stored online, I would recommend getting a physical record from time to time so that even if the doctor changes something within the system, you will have a hard copy to prove what has happened during your course of care.

Consider this: 41% of Americans have never even seen their medical record! That means that almost half the population is unaware of what is in their file! It's important to be clued into your own health and understand what is in your medical charts. It's also important to check for mistakes within your file. Doctors are human and do make mistakes, but imagine if they forgot to put an allergy down in your file or some other important piece of information that could be life-threatening? You want to make sure everything is up to date.

If my mother had requested her medical record after her first and second visit to her dermatologist, she would have had all the proof she needed to press charges against this negligent doctor. But because she waited too long to get a copy of her record, the doctor had a chance to change his notes and claim he had offered a biopsy and my mom refused it. Having doctors' notes and their course of treatment in writing in your hands is an immensely powerful tool. You can absolutely leverage this to your advantage. Doctors know that when there are other eyeballs on a medical record, it had better be accurate.

Many patients agree to go ahead with any treatment their doctor recommends. They have listened to their doctor's orders for so long that they don't even realize they have a choice in the matter.

One of the rights we have in our healthcare system is the right to make a treatment choice. As long as the patient is of sound mind, it is their right and responsibility to learn about the various treatment options for their condition and choose the option that best suits them.

Patients also have a right to informed consent. That means that any test, procedure, or treatment will only be performed after getting a signature from the patient acknowledging their consent. The practitioner is expected to explain the risks and benefits associated with the treatment option, although sometimes you may have to ask about these as the doctor may not offer this information upfront.

Patients also have the right to refuse treatment. This often happens at the end of life when patients wish to be comfortable instead of suffering through countless treatments meant to keep them alive. Sometimes, it comes down to the question of do you want more quality of life or more quantity of life? Patients also may refuse treatments proposed by their doctor in favor of alternative treatments, such as those with cancer. Just remember, you do not have to agree to go ahead with any test or procedure your doctor recommends.

Being assertive during doctor visits and hospital stays is crucial to getting the care you need. Patients and their caregivers who actively participate in their care have much better health outcomes than those who don't ask questions and just follow orders.

Assertiveness is not to be confused with aggressiveness, which will get you the opposite result you are looking for. Aggressive communication is hostile and demanding, while assertive communication is clear, concise, and confident. Assertive communication happens when needs and wishes are respectfully communicated while holding one's ground until the desired information is gotten and care received.

When being assertive, use "I" statements such as "I need to have my questions answered. I want to understand my condition. I will do what it takes to ensure the best treatment." Show empathy for the doctor or office worker by saying things like "I understand you are a very busy doctor, but it's very important that we discuss all of the treatment options before I can make a decision."

When your requests are ignored, you will need to become the squeaky wheel that gets the grease. You must be repetitive, stating the same thing over and over until you get what you want. Be insistent, persistent, consistent, clear, and concise!

Although you may have to blatantly stand up to a doctor or go and find another doctor, a beneficial patient/doctor relationship will involve both parties doing their part. You expect him/her to do their part, and you must also do your part. Keep a medical journal, including detailed notes of your condition. Do your own research, even printing out medical articles to show the doctor if they cannot figure out what's wrong and you have some ideas. Consider your doctor and you a team. Come to your appointment early and prepared with your medical information card, journal, research, and questions. Do not forget the recorder or pen and paper! Remember, there are way more patients than doctors and that will get worse in the future. So, be an active participant in your care.

CHAPTER 10

HOW TO APPEAL A DENIED CLAIM

Many people think when their insurance company denies their medical claim, that is the end of it. People fret about having to pay a massive bill on their own with no help from their insurance company. However, this is NOT the case. You can ALWAYS appeal a denied claim and you can even appeal your insurance company's decision to drop your coverage.

When your claim gets denied, your insurance company must tell you why they denied your claim and how you can dispute it. Ask your insurance company to do an internal review which requires them to do a full and fair review of its decision. If you are in a medical emergency, they are required to conduct this review faster. They must be able to fully explain why they denied your claim.

You also have the right to take your appeal to a third party for an external review. You can even opt for an external review first and skip the internal review process. Your insurance company must accept the decision of the third party, even if it means paying your claim. The third party gets the final say, either upholding the insurer's decision or appealing it in your favor.

To file an external review, you must file a written request within 4 months of receiving the denial of your claim. The types of claims that are eligible for external review are as follows:

- Any denial involving medical judgment. For example, if your doctor disagrees with the insurer's decision that a certain test is unnecessary
- Any denial based on the insurance company's judgment that the treatment is investigational or experimental
- If your coverage gets canceled based on a determination by your insurer that you falsified information on your application

Some states have Consumer Assistance Programs which are funded by federal grants. These programs help consumers with health insurance problems, helping them understand what their rights are and what they are entitled to through their health coverage. Consumer Assistance Programs also help consumers make informed decisions when choosing healthcare. If your state has a CAP, take advantage of this free service.

In all states, health insurance companies must offer an external review process that meets "Federal Consumer Protection Standards". This is a 16-page document published by the Department of Health and Human Services that goes into detail about the 16 minimum consumer protection standards. This document is accessible on healthcare.gov.

If your state has an external review process that meets or goes beyond the minimum standard, your insurer will be required to use the state's external review process. If your state does not have an external review process that meets the minimum standards, the Department of Health and Human Services run by the federal government will oversee an external review process.

In states where the federal government oversees the process, your insurance company can either use the Health and Human Services administered process or hire a third-party independent review organization. Your insurance company is responsible for paying the fees associated with hiring an independent third-party company. You will be charged <u>no more than $25 for this process</u>.

You can find the contact information for the company that will conduct your external review on your Explanation of Benefits (EOB) for your insurance company or on the final denial from your insurer after an internal review is conducted. Remember, you always have a right to an independent third-party external review at any time, even before asking for an internal review.

External reviews are conducted as soon as possible, and no later than 45 days after the appeal was submitted. In case of a medical emergency, such as an emergency surgery needed, external reviews must be conducted within 72 hours.

If you are ready to file a secure appeal, visit **externalappeal.cms.gov**. This portal is the best method for filing a claim. If you are not able to file this way, there are fax and mail options. There is also a form for someone else to file an appeal for you such as a doctor or health advocate.

On average, around half of people who appeal denied claims get the decision overturned in their favor. The problem is the vast majority of people do not even try to appeal their denied claim. Many people don't even know they can.

In the year 2017 alone, _42 million claims were denied_ by 121 major insurance companies. A Kaiser Family Foundation report found that only 0.05% (less than 200,000) of these denials were appealed! Even more shocking, only around 0.009% (1 in 11,000) of customers went directly to an external review, although everyone who has insurance has the right to bypass the internal review process in favor of an immediate external review.

Don't pass up any opportunity. If any medical claim gets denied, appeal it immediately! You have a 50/50 chance of getting it repealed, and even more in some states. You can find the information you need on the Department of Health and Human Services website.

Good record keeping on your part will help you expedite this process. If your doctor feels your insurance should cover something that they are refusing to cover, get them involved too.

If you cannot get your insurance to cover a diagnostic test, even after an external review, keep in mind that oftentimes the cash price of a test is much cheaper than the price the insurance companies are billed. If you want blood work, an MRI, or another type of test, ask for the cash deal price. You may be surprised to find that it is affordable enough to pay for these tests out of pocket rather than waiting for your condition to get bad enough to where the insurance companies would pay for these tests. Be proactive in your diagnostic and treatment plan. In some states they have programs based on wages. What I mean by that is they charge you for services based on what you make. In Colorado, it's called sunrise care. They even have dental services. So, if you get denied a procedure from your insurance company, start looking for these options in your state. My mother was able to get a grant through this service to fix her dental issues.

CHAPTER 11

HEALTHY LIVING AND STAYING OUT OF THE HOSPITAL

Oftentimes, medical care is used to treat problems that are already there. Rarely do doctors educate us about preventative measures we can take to stay out of the doctor's office or hospital. Even in school when we were growing up, there was little focus on health education. P.E. class was the closest we got to health education, and even that was more about movement than about nutrition or healthy lifestyle habits.

Learning about basic self-care is a great way to prevent illness and disease. I'll share with you a few basic habits you can start practicing that could extend your life and greatly improve your health.

Water: Start with the Most Basic

Does your doctor ever ask you how much water you drink on a daily basis? No? Most doctors don't. This is strange because dehydration can cause all sorts of issues—excess body weight, stress and depression, headaches, high blood pressure, and more.

Dr. Fereydoon Batmanghelidj, M.D. devoted his life to studying the effects of chronic dehydration on health and disease. Dr. B was born in Iran and studied medicine in Scotland and London. He studied under Alexander Fleming who shared the Nobel prize for the discovery of penicillin. After practicing medicine in the UK for a few years, he moved back to his home country Iran where he played a key role in the development of hospitals and medical clinics.

During the Iranian Revolution, Dr. Batmanghelidj was held as a political prisoner in Evin Prison for 2 years and 7 months. It was during this time that he discovered the power of water in curing disease. One night, he treated a fellow prisoner who was having debilitating peptic ulcer pain. Since Dr. B had no medications to give him, he instead had him drink 2 glasses of water. In less than 10 minutes, his pain was gone. The prisoner was instructed to drink 2 glasses of water every 3 hours and remained pain-free for the remainder of his 4-month stay in prison.

Dr. Batmanghelidj went on to successfully treat 3,000 prisoners who had stress induced peptic ulcer pain with water alone. At one point, Dr. B was offered an early release for his good deeds but decided to stay the remaining 4 months to continue helping other prisoners and studying their results. When his time in prison was up, he escaped Iran and moved to the United States where he continued his research on what he called "Chronic Unintentional Dehydration".

According to Dr. B, dry mouth is not a reliable indicator of dehydration. Through his studies, he found that chronic dehydration produces pain and many degenerative diseases including adult-onset diabetes, hypertension, arthritis, angina, asthma, lupus, and multiple sclerosis. He found that many diseases that doctors were treating with medication could actually be more effectively treated with water!

He authored a book titled "Your Body's Many Cries for Water" where he presents research and evidence to show that many illnesses are a direct result of unintentional chronic dehydration. His message to the world can be summed up in the book's tagline: "You are not sick, you are thirsty. Don't treat thirst with medication."

Before you run to your doctor, first try Dr. B's recommendation: drink half your body weight in ounces of water per day. So, for example, if you weigh 160 pounds, you will need to drink 80 ounces (about 2.37 L) of water over the course of one day. Make sure to keep some salt in your diet which will help your cells retain the water. This may seem like a lot of water initially, especially if you have been chronically dehydrated your whole life. Gradually increase your water intake until you are getting the proper amount.

Consider this: your blood is 82% water, your muscles are 75% water, your lungs are 90% water, your brain is 76% water, and even your bones are 25% water! Seeing these numbers, do you think that having a lack of water in your body could present some problems? It's obvious, right?

Water is a nearly free solution, yet doctors almost never educate their patients about the importance of proper hydration. Unfortunately, simple and cost-effective solutions don't make doctors and pharmaceutical companies money, so they don't necessarily have much motivation to advocate for these solutions.

Water should be your first treatment option used to improve your health. Get yourself a 32 oz bottle and carry it around with you throughout the day. Most people will need to drink 2-3 of these bottles per day. Having a water vessel with measurements on the side will help you track your intake. Replace soda and sugary drinks with water and you will notice your weight start to drop while your aches and pains begin to subside. You'll understand the power of proper hydration when you consistently stay hydrated and notice how much better you feel.

Diet: Thousands of Studies Confirm That Food Directly Affects Health

With all the new diets circulating, sometimes it can be confusing to tell what's healthy and what isn't. In fact, a recent study done by the International Food Information Council Foundation found that 80% of the population is confused about nutrition! Food fads circulate on social media, and some are based on facts while others are not. When we look at the science of how our food affects our health, researchers do agree on some basic nutritional guidelines.

Plants Should Rule Your Diet

An article titled "Nutritional Update for Physicians: Plant-Based Diets" posted on the US Institutes of Health National Library of Medicine says this: "Research shows that plant- based diets are cost-effective, low-risk interventions that may lower body mass index, blood pressure, HbA1C (blood glucose), and cholesterol levels. They may also reduce the number of medications needed to treat chronic diseases and lower ischemic heart disease mortality rates. *Physicians should consider recommending a plant-based diet to all their patients, especially those with high blood pressure, diabetes, cardiovascular disease, or obesity.*"

The health benefits of a plant-based diet have been

backed by research for decades, so why don't doctors teach their patients about this? The problem starts in medical school, where few doctors get any nutritional education. On average, only 1% of the lecture time students receive is about nutrition. Even this small amount of education does not place emphasis on the importance of a plant-based diet in disease prevention. Doctors can't teach their patients something they don't understand themselves.

A recent study published in the Oxford Academic's Journal of Nutrition measured biomarkers in people with various diets, from vegan to vegetarian to non-vegetarian. Biomarkers are substances in the body that are measured to obtain an objective state of health or disease in a patient. This year-long study involved 909 participants and was designed to examine how various diet patterns affect health outcomes. Levels of various biomarkers were obtained from blood, urine, and tissue samples.

The study found that vegans had the highest levels of healthy biomarkers that indicate resiliency and the lowest levels of unhealthy biomarkers that indicate disease. Vegetarians who ate some dairy, eggs, and/or fish had the second-best outcome. Non- vegetarians came in last with the lowest levels of healthy biomarkers and the highest levels of unhealthy biomarkers.

Plants provide phytonutrients, which have antioxidant and anti-inflammatory properties. They also boost immunity, detoxify carcinogens, and repair DNA damage. Plants provide us with a wide array of vitamins and minerals that we need to survive. Even the USDA recommends we fill 75% of our plates with plants!

In a PubMed article that reviewed 87 published studies, authors Berkow and Barnard reported that vegan and vegetarian diets are highly effective for weight loss. They also found that people who had adopted a vegetarian diet had lower blood pressure and decreased rates of heart disease, diabetes, and obesity.

While you don't need to adopt a strict vegan diet, you can improve your health by making plants the superstars of your meals. Instead of having meat with every meal, start finding plant-based recipes that you can integrate into your diet. Here are a few ideas: Start by swapping out your egg and cheese breakfast sandwich with oatmeal topped with fruit, nuts, cinnamon, and honey. For lunch, how about a colorful salad with garbanzo beans as the protein source? At dinnertime, a vegetarian chili can be just as satisfying without meat if you put the right seasonings, veggies, and beans in it.

As a growing body of research confirms that plants should be our primary food source, adoption of a plant-based lifestyle is getting more widespread. As a result, stores carry more vegan and vegetarian options, many offering plant-based substitutes for everything you could think of—cheese, yogurt, milk, and even meat. Millions of vegan and vegetarian recipes fill the internet, offering scrumptious alternatives to all of your favorite dishes.

Cultural stigmas towards reducing animal product

consumption prevent many from improving their health. The Standard American Diet is filled with burgers, steaks, and cheese. Unhealthy choices are everywhere and many pride themselves on being "meat- eating Americans". However, numbers don't lie. Scientific studies and statistics overwhelmingly point to plants as our key to maintaining health and longevity. I felt great when I transitioned to a vegetarian diet with limited meat consumption. When I eat red meat, I usually end up feeling awful and slow. I was at my fastest in my boxing career when I stuck to the vegetarian diet with lots of nuts.

Red Meat and Processed Meats Increase Risk of Disease

I know, I know the meat thing. But science proves it is true. Not all meats are created equal. Red meats (beef, lamb, pork) have been classified as a Group 2A carcinogen by the World Health Organization, which means they likely cause cancer. Processed meats such as hotdogs, bacon, ham, and salami are Group 1 carcinogens, meaning they are known to cause cancer based on strong scientific evidence.

A chemical in red meat called Heam is broken down in the gut to produce N-nitroso chemicals which have been found to damage cells that line the bowel. This can lead to colon cancer. Processed meats also produce this harmful chemical when broken down and the nitrates and nitrites used as preservatives in meat have the same harmful effect when digested.

A recent meta-analysis published in the National Institutes of Health Library of Medicine concludes that higher consumption of red meat and processed meats are associated with an increased risk of mortality from cardio-vascular disease, cancers, and other health complications.

Research presented by the European Society of Cardiology has alarming findings as well. In this observational study including nearly 20,000 participants, an increase in red and processed meat intake was associated with poorer heart function. Individuals who consumed more of these meats had stiffer arteries, smaller ventricles, and hearts that did not function as well. These individuals were also more likely to have high blood pressure, high cholesterol, diabetes, and obesity. Previous studies done on the topic found an increased risk of heart attacks and death from heart disease when consuming red and processed meats.

Studies have not found these same results with participants who ate poultry and fish. Poultry was not found to significantly increase the risk of heart disease and the essential fatty acids in fish have actually been found to *improve* heart and vascular health. If you want to keep meat in your diet, studies show better health outcomes when opting for poultry and fish over red and processed meats.

Harvard Medical School's Dr. Frank Hu says we don't

even need red meat in our diets to meet our nutritional requirements. Red meat's nutritional claim to fame is that it's high in protein, iron, B12, zinc, and selenium. We can get the same amount of these nutrients, if not more, from eating poultry, fish, eggs, and nuts. Following a balanced plant-based diet can also provide the proper amount of essential nutrients the body needs.

Choose Whole Foods Over Processed and Fast Foods

Processed foods line our supermarket shelves much like fast food chains line our streets. Processed food is EVERYWHERE. It may be more convenient and sometimes cheaper, but a steady diet of these toxic foods will put us in the fast lane to disease.

Processed foods tend to be full of sugar, corn syrup, salt, saturated fats, oils, artificial flavors, and preservatives. Heavy competition in the food industry encourages companies to create food that tastes better and is actually addicting to consumers. The food industry even puts a leavening agent called Azodicarbonamide (ACA) in our bread which is toxic and is linked to kidney and thyroid cancers! They originally used it to form bubbles in plastics and foam!!! This chemical is illegal in most other countries, even China! Why not here?!?

The main issue with these "convenience foods" is they

fill our bodies with toxins while failing to deliver nutrients and actually blocking the absorption of nutrients we need to stay healthy. While these foods satisfy your initial hunger and craving for fat, salt, and sugar, they will quickly leave you hungry again as your body never received the nutrition it required. Due to these foods' addictive nature, you will probably eat more of the same foods, adding to your body's toxic load yet still leaving you nutrient deficient.

Nature provides us with everything our bodies need. Foods like raw almonds, leafy greens, and apples each offer their own unique combination of vitamins, minerals, and other nutrients that humans simply can't replicate with man-made food. Stick to nature's medicine by eating foods that are unprocessed and as close to their original form as possible.

Another thing, NO MORE non-stick pans! They are created using PFAS (polyfluoroalkyl substances) which are extremely carcinogenic! People who own birds are told to take ALL non-stick pans out of the home, due to the toxins they give off while cooking. It will kill your bird dead because of the way their respiratory system is designed. If it does that to them, you know it's not good for us either. PFASs have been found in all water sources in the world now and are "forever chemicals" - seriously bad news! Protect your health by using normal pans for cooking.

Supplements Save Lives

Experts agree we are a nation that is overfed and undernourished. We favor quantity over quality, and as a result, an estimated 92% of the population is nutrient deficient in some way. Even if we make an effort to eat healthily, our nation's soil is so depleted due to corporate farming practices that even our produce is less nutrient dense than it used to be.

According to the CDC and the USDA:

- Over 50% of the population is Vitamin D deficient, with 90% of the African American population and 70% of the elderly population being Vitamin D deficient
- 90% of Americans are deficient in Potassium
- 80% are Vitamin E deficient
- 70% are Calcium deficient
- 50% of Americans are deficient in Vitamin A, Vitamin C, and Magnesium

There have always been debates in the medical field as to whether or not people need supplements, but an overwhelming amount of research has made this national issue very apparent. Even the American Medical Association, which once took a stance against supplementation, now advises all adults to take at least one whole food multivitamin every day. Make sure it doesn't contain fillers. There are quite a bit of crappy "vitamins" out there. In fact, it's a multi-billion-dollar business. So, do your research and get a good whole food vitamin. Talk to a nutritionist and get some recommendations.

Make sure you cover your nutritional bases by taking a supplement. You will be giving your body the tools it needs to function and heal while preventing a host of diseases that could cut your life short.

Exercise - Moving and Grooving Your Way to Health

Did I mention that I was a personal trainer at one point in my life too? I trained at Bally's Total Fitness, for those of you who remember them. Exercise is not optional if you want to stay healthy. In order to maintain health, it is essential to do some form of activity on a regular basis. According to the CDC (Center for Disease Control and Prevention), regular physical activity reduces the risk of chronic diseases like type 2 diabetes, dementia, depression, anxiety, many types of cancer, and heart disease.

Exercise isn't just about preventing disease, though. It's also about improving the quality of your life and your mental health. Regular exercise improves mood and energy levels while decreasing depression and anxiety. It also helps you sleep better, allowing the body to heal more quickly and efficiently.

CDC guidelines recommend 150 minutes of moderate aerobic activity every week in addition to strength training at least 2 times per week. You don't necessarily need a gym membership to stay healthy, though. In fact, walking is one of the best full body activities you can do. Going on 30-minute walks 5 days a week will get you to 150 minutes of aerobic activity. And for strength training? Consider 15–20-minute YouTube videos focused on building muscle. When using your own body weight to strength train, as with pushups, sit-ups, and squats, you don't even need to buy equipment like dumbbells or straps. Keep it simple to build habits that last.

The key to staying motivated with exercise is finding something you absolutely love to do. Not everyone wants to be a gym rat, spending hours in a loud sweaty room with other people. For those who are nature lovers, hiking and climbing are great ways to stay in shape while enjoying the outdoors. For people who love music, dancing can be a fun way to stay fit. A study done by Science Journal stated that the elderly who participated in dancing with a group of people had less Dementia/Alzheimer's and were happier overall. Some love the discipline and community aspect of learning a martial art and thrive in this environment. Did you do a sport in high school that you really loved? Find a community league and get back in the game!

The point is this: to build lasting habits, you need to find something that you genuinely enjoy and want to keep doing day after day, year after year. Exercise doesn't need to be a chore. You can combine it with one of your hobbies and turn it into the best part of your day that you always look forward to. Not only will you be healthier for it, but you'll be happier too, and your quality of life will greatly improve.

Stress Reduction and Mental Health Care

Humans and animals have a built-in stress response that helps us stay alive. This stress response is part of the sympathetic nervous system which enables us to deal with an immediate threat through fighting or flighting. Short-term stress is positive in that it prepares the body for action, keeps it alert, and improves immune response. However, the key phrase is "short-term". When you observe an animal after dealing with a stressful situation, they will literally shake it off, releasing the stress through some type of movement, and then go about their day.

In our fast-paced society, stressors are a constant part of our lives. Traffic, bills, work, relationships, and over-stimulation from television and the internet keeps most of us in a constant state of stress. This type of chronic stress has been shown to decrease immune system function by raising suppressor T-cell and cortisol levels, making us more susceptible to getting viral infections, and can lead to adrenal fatigue.

Chronic stress also alters acid levels in the stomach, which can lead to peptic ulcers, stomach ulcers, and ulcerative colitis. Stress leads to histamine release, which can worsen asthma and allergy symptoms. When stress is not managed, more serious psychiatric illnesses can manifest. Many studies have linked chronic stress to the onset of major depressive disorder, psychosis, bipolar disorder, and PTSD.

Stress is not just a problem in your mind, it has detrimental effects on your physical health too. For this reason, managing your stress is hugely important in staying healthy. Here is a list of activities that are scientifically proven to reduce your stress and bring balance to the mind and body:

- Exercise
- Yoga
- Meditation
- Social support from friends
- Deep breathing
- Talk Therapy
- Massage therapy

Exercise is a fantastic way to reduce stress on a daily basis and release some "feel good" chemicals called endorphins into your brain.

Another wonderful way to reduce stress is by relaxing your muscles (ever notice how tense you are when sitting in traffic or arguing with someone?). You can do this by taking a hot bath or shower, getting a massage, and stretching. Experts have also proven that deep breathing reduces the stress of the moment. Trust me, try it, it works. Many studies have demonstrated how yoga can help to reduce and manage stress, anxiety, and depression. Yoga incorporates deep breathing into a stretching and strengthening routine, which also calms the mind and regulates brain function.

Instead of getting caught up in a society that pressures us into going a million miles per hour, go against the grain and decrease stress by slowing down. Leave for work and appointments early so you can enjoy the drive without rushing.

Drive in the slow lane to avoid road rage drivers speeding down the freeway. Shifting your life out of the fast lane and cultivating peace is a challenging but worthwhile pursuit.

CHAPTER 12

BE OPEN TO ALTERNATIVE TREATMENTS

There will probably come a time when you will need to seek treatment outside of the western medical system. Sometimes the doctor is unable to come to a diagnosis or find a problem with the diagnostic tools he/she has. Many people get frustrated after having several appointments with specialists, only to be told that nothing seems to be wrong or that it's all in their head.

As we talked about before, it's particularly important to trust your gut and trust the messages your body is sending you. Don't let the doctors de-legitimize your symptoms just because they are unable to find the problem. Seeking alternative treatments will give you another perspective using a different system of diagnostics.

It's ironic that we call systems of medicine like acupuncture and herbology "alternative" because many of them were around long before western medicine was. Our medical system often looks down on these treatments and considers them "snake oil" medicine although many doctors don't even know how these systems work.

Remember, very few doctors are educated about nutrition in medical school. The tools they are given for treatment are drugs and surgery. Unfortunately, medical schools do not teach doctors to take a holistic and well-rounded approach, but instead, encourage separating the parts of the individual and treating them independently.

For example, Traditional Chinese Medicine considers the emotional state of the patient when diagnosing and treating any condition. In Western medicine, you are either treated for a physical or a psychological condition, but rarely does the same doctor consider both aspects of your being.

While modern medicine is absolutely incredible in treating life-threatening conditions and prolonging life in the midst of disease, rarely is the focus on prevention through lifestyle choices. It's important to understand the limitations of modern medicine when seeking solutions to your health problems. Be open to trying a variety of treatments before you give up hope of finding a solution.

Consult a Nutritionist and Food Allergy Testing

Researchers have found that 70% of strokes, 70% of colon cancers, 80% of coronary artery disease, and 90% of type 2 diabetes are preventable by _following a healthy diet_, not smoking, moderate exercise, and limiting alcohol consumption.

Americans suffer from diseases of malnutrition and excess. We are getting too many of the foods we don't need (excess sugars, salts, oils, and preservatives) and not enough of the nutrients we do need. We are getting too many of the things that harm us and not enough of the nutrients that help us.

According to the Centers for Disease Control, 9 out of 10 Americans have too much sodium in their diets. 1 in 4 Americans eat some sort of fast food every day. Even sadder still, Americans consume 31% _more_ packaged food than fresh food. _Less than 10% of adults and adolescents are getting enough fruits and veggies._ It doesn't help that the cost of food is ridiculous these days. The reason for this is all the food is owned by only three companies, another reason to become politically active. Try farmers' markets. They tend to be cheaper and healthier options.

What you put in your mouth every day is the greatest contributor to health or disease in your body and mind. Because doctors are not educated in the realm of nutrition and how diet relates to disease, they often have no recommendations for changes in your diet.

Diseases that have been linked to a poor diet include:

- Osteoarthritis
- Heart disease
- Coronary Artery Disease
- Stroke
- Many Types of Cancers
- Sleep Apnea
- Gallbladder Disease
- Obesity
- Asthma
- Insulin Resistance
- Depression and Anxiety
- Digestive Health Issues
- Type 2 Diabetes
- Dementia and Alzheimer's
- Respiratory Issues
- Tooth Decay
- Fatty liver
- Fatigue

People are confused about what a healthy diet is. A recent survey revealed that people find doing their taxes less complicated than trying to figure out how to eat healthily. With all the mixed messages on the internet about which diet is the healthiest, seeking the advice of a professional can get you answers and solutions to your specific problem.

Find a nutritionist to address your specific needs

You may consider food allergy testing to get proof that certain foods are having adverse reactions to your health. The nutritionist will help you formulate a diet plan that works best for your body. Some people are lactose intolerant or gluten intolerant and don't even know it until they get a test. When they eliminate these things from their diets, suddenly their energy comes back, skin clears up, and other health issues get better with this slight dietary change.

It's extremely important to give your body the best chance at healing and survival by keeping it properly hydrated (with half your body weight in ounces per day) and by eating a healthy, balanced diet full of whole, organic, unprocessed foods (like vegetables, fruits, grains, lean meats, legumes, and herbs). As organic foods have become more popular for people to buy, corporations have jumped on the bus. Many of these are labeled "organic" but don't be fooled. Do your research to ensure you're getting truly organic foods. A good indicator is the label USDA-CERTIFIED ORGANIC!

A nutritionist can help you find the right supplements

and herbs for your needs as well. Yearly blood work will show deficiencies and excesses that need to be addressed. Following the advice of professionals who have studied the science behind nutrition for many years will yield incredible results. By being conscious of your dietary choices, you will give your body the absolute best chance of healing.

Choosing Super Star Supplements

In the last chapter, we talked about the importance of taking a daily multivitamin to cover all of your nutritional bases. When doing so, it's important that your supplement be derived from whole foods. Whole food supplements are easier for the body to digest and absorb while providing additional phytonutrients. These supplements should preferably be organic. Make sure there are no fillers in your supplement. Harmful fillers include:

- Titanium dioxide (can cause cancers)
- Magnesium stearate (inhibits nutrient absorption)
- Hydrogenated oils (increases bad cholesterol)
- Artificial colors (for example: red #40 and blue #2 can cause cancer)
- Artificial flavors (hard for the body to process)
- PCBs, lead, and mercury (often found in fish oils due to ocean contamination)

Make sure your supplement is not harming you with the toxic fillers in it. These fillers are meant to aid in processing and help the supplement look and taste better, making it more appealing to consumers. However, these fillers make the supplement hard for the body to absorb and process. An organic, plant-based whole food supplement with no extra ingredients or sugars is best.

A good example of a vitamin that has good intentions but is actually harming people is fish oil. Many people take fish oil to get their omegas which contribute to brain health, eye health, heart health, cancer prevention, and more. The thing most people don't know is that the gel capsules are often heat sealed. When you heat fish oil it becomes rancid and not only useless nutritionally, but is also somewhat harmful.

Also, due to micro-plastics and ocean toxicity from nuclear spills such as the one that happened in Fukushima in 2011, *fish are extremely contaminated. **Japan plans to release more than 100 million tons of contaminated water into the ocean from its destroyed nuclear plant over the next several years.** **<u>If you haven't switched to plant-based omegas yet, the time is now</u>**.

Plant based omegas like chia seeds, flax seeds, hemp seeds, pomegranate seeds, olive oil, seaweed, and edamame can give you all the omegas you need while providing other phytonutrients as well. If you don't think you are getting enough through your diet, consider a plant-based supplement like "The Omega Blend" from Juice Plus+.

It concentrates the power of raspberry seeds, buckthorn berries, algae, safflower seeds, pomegranate seeds, and tomato seeds. It is sealed without heat and protected from oxidation using nitrogen filled capsules. These nutrient dense plants and algae provide omegas 3, 5, 6, 7, and 9 - a complete blend that supports vision, brain function, and heart health.

As far as other whole foods supplements go, Registered Dietician Nutritionist Cynthia Wigutow who is a board-certified specialist in oncology and dietetics recommends the following herbs for cancer prevention:

- Turmeric (anti-inflammatory, inhibits cancer cell growth)
- Ginger (antioxidant, anti-inflammatory, appetite stimulant)
- Cayenne Pepper (toxic to cancer cells, helps prevent cancer growth)
- Saffron (inhibits tumor growth and cancer progression)
- Oregano (the richest source of antioxidants amongst the herbs, promotes cancer cell death)
- Garlic (the most powerful anti-cancer plant, garlic helps fight disease and prevents growth of cancer cells)

What are some other helpful plants that have potent effects on the body?

Mushrooms for Enhanced
Immune System Function

In a meta-analysis of observational studies, an increase in mushroom consumption has been associated with a lower risk of all types of cancer, especially breast cancer. Mushrooms such as maitake, shiitake, and button mushrooms increase immune system function and even have anti-tumor and anti-cancer properties.

A mushroom extract known as AHCC was formulated in Japan in 1987 by extracting and concentrating the healing properties of cultured shiitake mushrooms. It has been shown to improve immune system function, increasing natural killer cells, promoting macrophage and T-cell activity, and increasing dendritic cell activity. This all equates to giving the body a bigger, better, stronger army to fight off infections and disease.

AHCC has been studied extensively by hospitals and universities around the world for over 20 years because of its promising results in the prevention and treatment of colds, flues, cancers, cardiovascular diseases, hepatitis, diabetes, and viruses such as HPV. In one study, half of the participants who were taking AHCC daily were able to put their HPV infections into remission within 6 months.

AHCC not only helps the body fight and kill cancer cells, but it also helps to protect the body during chemotherapy and radiation, decreasing symptoms and strengthening bones and tissues. Patients taking AHCC also showed a longer postoperative survival rate after having cancer removed.

Many supplements are becoming available to help people get more mushrooms into their diets. The most potent medicinal mushrooms include:

- Shiitake
- Maitake
- Chaga
- Reishi
- Cordyceps
- Lion's Mane
- Agaricus
- Poria

Seek out supplements that give you a variety of mushrooms or a highly concentrated version such as in the case of AHCC. Mushrooms give the immune system a well- rounded boost as they increase innate immunity and adaptive immunity, launching generalized and specific attacks on invaders.

CBD for Anxiety, Seizures, Pain Relief, and More

Since CBD became legal in all 50 states in 2018, more people have been finding the amazing therapeutic effects of this cannabinoid. CBD doesn't have psychoactive effects like THC, but does provide relief from nausea, anxiety, inflammation, and pain. It can also help regulate sleep and appetite and works well for symptom relief during chemotherapy and radiation.

In 1992, the first endocannabinoid was discovered in the human brain. Since then, cannabinoid receptors have been found in many parts of the body including the central nervous system, immune system, digestive tract, and reproductive organs. The endocannabinoid system is intimately connected with our state of health. This system helps to regulate and maintain balance within the body's vital systems.

Our own bodies make cannabinoids, however some people don't make enough, as discovered in cannabinoid deficiency syndrome. Some conditions that are linked to Clinical Endocannabinoid Deficiency (CED) are fibromyalgia, migraines, and irritable bowel syndrome. Conditions such as these that are treatment-resistant to pharmaceuticals often respond well to a CBD supplement. It is thought that when the body receives enough cannabinoids, it is able to bring itself back into homeostasis.

Since hemp in all of its forms has been illegal for many years and was only legalized recently in 2018, there have been few well-conducted trials that give substantial evidence to the benefits of CBD. However, shortly after hemp was legalized, the FDA approved a drug called Epidiolex which uses CBD as its active ingredient to treat seizures in those who have epilepsy. CBD has been shown in several studies to reduce the frequency of seizures by almost 44% in most participants.

Animal studies have shown promising results with pain relief using CBD. Cannabidiol reduces inflammation and acts on the pain sensing pathways to reduce pain. Canada has approved a treatment that uses a 1:1 THC and CBD medication to relieve patients of central nerve related pain such as multiple sclerosis and cancer pain that proved unresponsive to optimized opioid therapy.

When applied topically, CBD can provide relief from arthritis along with other joint and muscle inflammation. It penetrates into the tissues, reducing inflammation and pain with no side effects. I use CBD every day on my back to eliminate pain and muscle spasms. Friends of mine who have tried it have told me that it's "better than Advil". I've had such positive effects with it that I always keep some in my purse and use it daily.

A laboratory study found that CBD also prevents sebocytes from producing too much sebum, which can cause acne. Applied topically, CBD can help improve complexion by reducing inflammation and preventing future breakouts.

There is much anecdotal evidence from people claiming that CBD helped them manage their anxiety and depression. While the exact mechanism is unknown, CBD is thought to have a positive effect on serotonin levels (the happy chemical) in the brain. CBD also interacts with the receptors that control addiction, appetite, and nausea.

In a case study of 72 participants, 48 of them (66.7%)

reported an improvement in sleep scores in the first month of use. In a separate study, 31% of patients who started taking CBD for other symptoms such as pain or inflammation reported sleeping better as well. Preliminary research suggests that CBD can help with insomnia, REM sleep behavior disorder, and chronic daytime sleepiness. By balancing your sleep cycles, you will get more restful sleep and be more awake and alert during the day.

Several small studies have shown promising evidence in improving the quality of life for patients with Parkinson's, Diabetes, Cancers, PTSD, MS, Opioid Addiction, Lupus, and other life-altering conditions. Continue to do your own research as more studies reveal the health benefits of CBD and other cannabinoids.

Rick Simpson Oil Harnesses the Entourage Effect

Also known as RSO, Rick Simpson Oil is a full spectrum concentrate made from the entire cannabis plant. This thick, resin-like substance is filled with a variety of cannabinoids and terpenes. It was first created by a Canadian named Rick Simpson who was an engineer that got injured at work while removing asbestos from a hospital boiler room. He was knocked unconscious by the fumes and suffered dizziness and ringing in the ears (tinnitus) for many years after the incident.

No pharmaceuticals were helping Rick Simpson, so he decided to take matters into his own hands by trying alternative solutions. He heard about marijuana's medicinal benefits for conditions such as seizures and thought it might help him. He started growing and using the plant and was able to alleviate his dizziness and tinnitus symptoms with the use of marijuana.

Years later, Rick was diagnosed with basal cell carcinoma, a form of skin cancer. After reading a study published in The Journal of the National Cancer Institute about THC killing cancer cells in mice, Rick was motivated to try using THC on his own skin cancer.

He made a highly concentrated extract and applied it to his carcinoma. Within a week the spot was gone.

After having such incredible success with this plant, Rick Simpson spread the word and taught others how to make this highly potent concentrate. He never patented his extraction method because he wanted it to be available to as many people as possible. Friends and neighbors of his were able to reverse their late-stage cancers (internally and externally) and treat other ailments as well.

"The entourage effect" is the theory that marijuana compounds work better together than individually. Full spectrum extracts are thought to be so effective because cannabinoids, terpenes, fatty acids, flavonoids, and phenols are maintained during extraction. Learn more about Rick Simpson and his full spectrum extract by watching the free documentary "Run From the Cure" on YouTube.

If this is your last resort, what the heck, you might as well try it. What do you have to lose?

RSO for Ulcerative Colitis and IBS

My friend's boyfriend has suffered from ulcerative colitis for about 10 years. He had stabilized his condition through prescription medication but never really got rid of the condition completely. He would still have flare-ups from time to time which made his girlfriend seek alternative solutions.

They cleaned up their diet, stayed active through exercising, and made sure to drink plenty of water every day. When my friend was searching around on YouTube for alternative solutions for ulcerative colitis, she came across a video about Rick Simpson Oil. The guy in the video claimed that after no medication could cure him, he found RSO. He began using it and after a month his colitis started clearing up. After 6 months, he had no symptoms at all.

My friend decided to have her boyfriend try taking it every night or every other night for a few months. After about a year of using it on and off, it was time for her boyfriend to get his regular colonoscopy done to check on his condition. Directly after the procedure, medical staff said that everything looked normal. My friend didn't really understand what this meant since her boyfriend's condition was not normal. They decided to wait for the doctor to call them and give them more detailed information.

When the doctor called, he sounded confused. "I don't really see any signs of colitis anymore. I guess we can say that it's in remission." Everybody was shocked by the outcome. Along with a healthy lifestyle, the RSO had worked! They never thought he could even be cured of this condition. By seeking solutions outside of the medical system, they found something that seemed like a miracle, fixing a condition that modern medicine claims there is no cure for. Anecdotal evidence suggests that RSO could help with other chronic bowel conditions such as IBS.

Niacin-amide for Skin Cancer

I first found out about Niacin-amide from a Lassen's store worker who also happened to be a retired rocket engineer. When I asked if they had any supplements that would help prevent skin cancer, he told me about Niacin-amide right away. He had found out about it from a customer who had been cut on 18 times for skin cancer. This customer was having skin cancer occurrences about every 3 months. His nutritionist told him to start taking 1000 mg of Niacin-amide every day and within 6 months he stopped getting skin cancer formations. Every 6-month follow-up after that confirmed clear and healthy skin.

I had previously been cut on 3 times for skin cancer and I knew I was prone to it as it runs in my family. My mother had the same problem where she was starting to get cut on every 6 months. I didn't want to keep having surgeries and I knew there had to be another way. I decided to try Niacin-amide, a concentrated complex B3 supplement. I took the same amount as the customer I was told about - 1000 mg per day.

Sure enough, I was another success story. Within a month I noticed not only was my skin clearing up from pre-cancerous spots, but my complexion was improving and even my hair and nails looked better and grew faster. At my six month checkup with a dermatologist, she gave me a clean bill of health. No skin cancer to be found. Every 6-month checkup since then has proven to have the same results - healthy, clear skin.

My mom experienced the same thing. She was the one who had terrible cancer on her nose that caused half of it to be taken off. She was starting to get skin cancer regularly, but since starting to take Niacin-amide she hasn't had a cancer incidence since. She also told a friend of hers about it and helped her prevent any more cancer spots and surgeries as well. I've helped at least 3 people that I know prevent further cancerous growths on their skin using the same treatment regimen: <u>1000 mg of Niacin-amide every day</u>.

I know this powerful supplement helps with more than skin cancer. Two friends of mine were able to cut their rosacea symptoms in half while taking Niacin-amide.

Funny thing is some hospitals don't even want nurses

to share this information. I remember telling a patient about Niacin-amide who came in for something completely unrelated. I noticed he had gotten surgery on his face, and I asked him what had happened. "Skin cancer" was his reply. He was healing but I saw a chance for prevention in the future and told him about the potent supplement that had helped me so much. Later, I was reprimanded by my boss and told that I shouldn't recommend any form of treatment to my patients. Strange, because that is completely within my scope of practice. Nurses tend to be better about recommending diet plans and supplements as they often know more about these things than doctors. (Nurses get more nutrition training in school than doctors do).

Unfortunately, my employer did not want to put patient care first and instead acted out of fear, telling me not to share my life-saving knowledge with my patients. What a sick place that was. I even asked my dermatologist if she knew about Niacin-amide. She did. "Why didn't you recommend it to me?!" was my exasperated reply.

"I guess I didn't think about it," was her response.

Strange how in the medical system solutions that are non-pharmaceutical but can be just as effective if used early, are rarely mentioned by doctors. Permanent cures mean less money for doctors, hospitals, and pharmaceutical companies and are therefore not taught about or recommended.

Vitamin D for Disease Prevention

Are you someone who tends to get every cold going around? Are you sick WAY too often and wonder why? You are highly likely Vitamin D deficient just like the other 50-90% of Americans who lack Vitamin D. During the height of the Covid-19 pandemic, patients were tested for D levels. A study out of Spain revealed that 80% of severely ill COVID-19 patients in the ICU were Vitamin D deficient.

The reason comes from how Vitamin D reacts in the body. This fat-soluble steroid hormone plays a key role in immune system function, increasing production of immune cells and decreasing harmful inflammation. Vitamin D also binds to receptor sites, signaling genes to turn on or off. This can inhibit tumor growth and other virus multiplication. Deficiency can be linked to auto-immune disorders such as multiple sclerosis, rheumatoid arthritis, type 1 diabetes, certain cancers, and dementia.

Vitamin D originally gained notoriety in treating rickets - a condition directly caused by a deficiency of D where bones become soft and malleable, often causing bowed legs. Since Vitamin D is needed for calcium absorption, and calcium is needed for strong bones, rickets was able to be cured by supplementing with Vitamin D. To prevent bone loss and resulting conditions such as osteoporosis and fractures, supplement with D every day.

Vitamin D is most easily absorbed sublingually (under the tongue). Since most of the nutrient content is lost during digestion, aim to get your Vitamin D directly into your bloodstream. By either using a tincture or a dissolvable tablet under the tongue, this crucial vitamin can be absorbed quickly. During the initial stages of COVID, doctors didn't have a treatment, so they recommended people take vitamins D, C, and zinc.

Ashwagandha for Fertility

Often used in Ayurvedic Medicine (the traditional medical system of India even older than Chinese medicine), Ashwagandha means "smell of the horse" in Sanskrit. It is an herb that enhances strength, energy levels, and concentration.

As an adaptogen, Ashwagandha helps to counteract the effects of stress in the body, enhancing relaxation and reducing anxiety. Participants in a study done on the effects of this plant showed those who took ashwagandha slept significantly better and had much lower levels of cortisol than those who did not.

Ashwagandha may improve athletic performance, proven to increase muscle gain during strength training and increase oxygen absorption in the body.

This helpful herb has also been shown to reduce inflammation markers in the body. A recent study on COVID-19 patients showed that inflammation was significantly reduced over a 7-day period while taking 0.5 grams of Ashwagandha per day.

True to its name, the "smell of the horse" herb increases testosterone levels and fertility in men. Over an 8-week period, participants in a study who were taking Ashwagandha had a 14.7% increase in testosterone levels and an 18% increase in DHEA-S (a sex hormone involved in testosterone production). Sperm concentration and volume also greatly improved.

Moringa for many Conditions

Grown most abundantly in India, Moringa is a potent, nutrient-dense plant that is used to treat almost any condition you can think of. It has seen success in treating diabetes, cancer, ulcers, chronic inflammation, cardiovascular disease, arthritis, and other serious conditions.

The leaves, flowers, stems, bark, roots, and pods of the moringa tree all have health benefits. However, the dried moringa leaf and leaf powder provide the densest amount of nutrients. Moringa leaves are an abundant source of calcium, iron, potassium, magnesium, zinc, copper, phosphorus, protein, fiber, vitamin A, vitamins B1-3, vitamin C, and vitamin E!

Moringa can grow in tropical and sub-tropical regions throughout the world and is easy to cultivate, requiring little care. It is a great remedy for malnutrition, being grown and harvested in places like Africa to improve the health of impoverished people. Filled with a complete array of amino acids, an abundance of antioxidants, and a very balanced dose of just about all the vitamins and minerals you need, you get a lot of bang for your buck with Moringa.

Consider these facts to give you an idea of just how nutrient-dense this miracle plant is. Moringa provides per serving:

- 17 times more calcium than milk
- 9 times more protein than yogurt
- 7 times more vitamin C than oranges
- 10 times more vitamin A than carrots
- 15 times more potassium than bananas
- and 25 times more iron than spinach!

Studies have shown Moringa to improve both type 1 and type 2 diabetes. Moringa's insulin-like proteins regulate blood sugar levels in the body.

Moringa leaves, stems, and pods all have anti-cancer and anti-tumor properties, making it an awesome addition to any cancer treatment protocol.

I know of at least 3 people who got incredible arthritis relief from using Moringa. I'm talking about a drastic reduction in pain and inflammation to the point where their symptoms were nearly gone.

Other conditions that get better with the use of Moringa include cardiovascular disease, chronic inflammatory conditions, and bacterial/viral/fungal infections.

Chlorophyll

I was able to reverse my anemia and improve hemoglobin levels in my blood just by using chlorophyll. Hemoglobin is a protein that is essential to building red blood cells. Chlorophyll is molecularly similar to hemoglobin and thus helps the body produce more oxygen-carrying red blood cells. For this reason, conditions such as anemia and thalassemia can be reversed by getting enough chlorophyll in the body.

Chlorophyll is the pigment that gives plants their green color. Alfalfa, spinach, and wheatgrass are particularly high in chlorophyll. Since most people don't get enough of this incredibly important compound, chlorophyll supplements are available in liquid, powder, and capsule form, providing a concentrated, high dosage formula.

Chlorophyll is also well known for decreasing bad breath and body odor. It has skin healing properties, often having positive effects on healing acne. In addition, chlorophyll is a powerful antioxidant, preventing oxidative damage to cells which in turn prevents many types of cancer.

I used chlorophyll when I was competing at the Olympic trials in Colorado for boxing. It was a completely legal supplement since it is just a concentrated version of what a plant naturally has. I knew I would have a disadvantage because I was training at sea level in Hollywood California and competing at 5,000 feet against women training at that altitude with the current Olympic team. I had blood drawn before taking the supplement and then after. I went from 14.5 to 16.6 and outpaced the other fighters at the competition. It takes about 3 weeks to take effect. So, don't expect an immediate response.

Aloe Vera for Gut Healing

We usually think of sunburns when we think about aloe vera, but this is only part of the healing story of this versatile plant. Aloe vera was researched heavily by the government when nuclear power was invented. They found that aloe had success in treating thermal and radiation burns. As a result, the FDA approved the use of aloe vera cream in 1959 for over-the-counter treatment of burn conditions on the skin.

Aloe vera can help alleviate constipation as well as improving ulcers throughout the digestive tract. Aloe acts as a prebiotic, feeding healthy bacteria in the gut to help it flourish. It also has compounds that fight inflammation in the gut, which is why it can help with ulcers, colitis, and leaky gut syndrome.

In many parts of the world, aloe vera is used as a traditional remedy for diabetes mellitus. Studies suggest aloe can alleviate hyperglycemia and balance lipid profiles, preventing cardiovascular complications related to the disease. Containing an impressive 20 essential amino acids out of 22 that our body needs (along with other essential vitamins and minerals) aloe vera juice is gladly welcomed by the body for health and healing.

Probiotics for Intestinal Balance

The human gut is home to 100 trillion microorganisms! Among these microbes, there are nearly 1,000 distinct species of bacteria that live in the gut. Some bacteria are helpful such as those that fight inflammation. Some are harmful such as those that cause inflammation and disease. When the gut biome has a plentiful variety of beneficial bacteria, health is maintained. When the gut biome has less variety of healthy bacteria and more variety of bad bacteria, health problems arise.

Gut health is directly related to our diet. Consuming too many processed foods, refined sugars, fast foods, and alcohol can throw our gut health out of whack. Antibiotics are also notorious for causing an imbalance of gut bacteria as they kill both the good and the bad. So how do you know if your gut bacteria are out of balance? Some symptoms include:

- Excess gas
- Diarrhea
- Constipation
- Stomach cramps/pain
- Heartburn
- IBS (irritable bowel syndrome)

- Crohn's and Colitis (inflammatory bowel disease)
- SIBO (small intestine bacterial overgrowth)
- GERD (gastroesophageal reflux disease)
- Skin issues like acne
- Brain fog

Even mental health issues like anxiety and depression have been linked to poor gut health because the neurotransmitters in the brain are constantly communicating with the gut. In fact, a whopping 90% of our serotonin receptors live in our gut tissue. If there is an imbalance in the gut, expect an imbalance in mental health as well.

To maintain a balanced microbiome, first we need to understand prebiotics and probiotics. Prebiotics are plant fibers found in fruits and vegetables. They act as a fertilizer, encouraging the growth of healthy bacteria in the gut. Probiotics are strains of living organisms that directly add healthy bacteria to your gut biome such as those found in yogurt and kombucha. By eating the right foods (prebiotics and probiotics) and minimizing junk food, you can balance the delicate ecosystem that lives inside you.

Examples of great prebiotic sources include apples, bananas, oatmeal, onions, garlic, asparagus, leeks, spinach, blueberries, chia seeds, and flax seeds. Some great sources of probiotics include kimchi, sauerkraut, miso soup, kefir, sourdough bread, buttermilk, and tempeh.

In addition to cleaning up your diet, adding a probiotic supplement to your health regimen for a period of time can bring your gut health back into balance. Ingesting a high dose of probiotics is also helpful while taking antibiotics so you can restore the healthy bacteria in your gut. But check with your pharmacist before taking a dairy probiotic when on an antibiotic. Drugs like Cipro can't be mixed with dairy.

Along with ensuring you are taking clean supplements with no harmful fillers, also make sure the supplements you take are compatible with your prescription medication. For example, K2 is a vitamin that enhances the blood's ability to clot. If you are taking a blood thinner, you obviously don't want to help your body's clotting abilities. It's a good idea to do your research and consult your doctor before starting a new supplement as there may be a contradiction with your medication.

Getting as many nutrients from fresh, unprocessed food as you can is ideal. However, the rise of corporate farming has resulted in our soil being depleted of nutrients. The food we grow in America today is significantly less nutrient-rich than the food grown 100 years ago. As such, most people are deficient in some vitamins and minerals. It is in our best interest to take a whole food supplement to fill in the nutritional gaps.

Give yourself the best access to nutrient-dense foods by shopping at your local farmers' markets. Typically, local farmers are more educated about crop rotation and how to build rich, nutritious soil for healthy plants to grow in. Buy organic to decrease your exposure to toxic pesticides.

Chiropractic Care

Through hands-on manipulation of the spine and other joints of the body, chiropractic care aims to increase mobility and blood flow, encouraging the body to heal itself.

Around 22 million Americans seek chiropractic care every year. It is often the first go-to for back pain, neck pain, and musculoskeletal injury recovery. While this treatment is not appropriate for everyone, many do receive tremendous benefits from it.

I had an issue myself that doctors couldn't seem to treat. I was having pain down the back of my leg that was making it hard to walk. My primary physician couldn't find anything on the MRI and didn't know what to do except prescribe me muscle relaxers and pain pills. I knew there had to be an underlying reason for my pain and decided to seek alternative care.

My friend introduced me to a chiropractor who discovered that my sciatica was caused by misalignment in my pelvis, which radiated up my spine. Through a series of adjustments, ultrasound, red light laser, massage to break up scar tissue, and stretching, I was able to walk pain-free within 3 sessions.

I had a co-worker that was having a similar issue. She was getting the run around by her doctors as well. Same crap - pain meds, physical therapy, etc. with no effect at all. I gave her some of my topical CBD oil, which she said worked better than the pain medications, and sent her to my chiropractor. Within 1 session she had significant relief from pain and after 2 sessions, almost full recovery.

Traditional Chinese Medicine

Originating thousands of years ago, TCM (Traditional Chinese Medicine) is one of the oldest medical systems used to diagnose, prevent, and treat disease. Its goal is to create balance in the body between the opposing forces of Yin and Yang. Qi (the body's vital life force energy) flows through meridians (channels in the body) and blockages of this Qi can result in disease and imbalance. Traditional Chinese Medicine uses acupuncture, cupping, moxibustion, herbs, exercise, meditation, diet, and massage to restore balance and clear blockages in the body so Qi can flow freely. While many of you may think this is hokey, think about how long many of these Asian cultures live! A LOT longer than Caucasian cultures and they are often way healthier too!

Stem Cell Therapy

Stem cells are the original raw cell material of the body. They are basically blank slates that can turn into any of the 200 different cells our bodies need. These undifferentiated cells are most prevalent in the early embryonic developmental stage. As the embryo quickly grows into a fetus, it needs all the stem cells it can get to make new bones, muscles, tissues, and organs.

As we age, our bodies still have stem cells mainly in the bone marrow and fat. We have much fewer of these stem cells and they can't differentiate with as much variety as embryonic cells. This is why we don't regenerate and heal as quickly when we get older. The fewer stem cells, the slower our body can create specialized cells that it needs.

French oncologist Georges Mathe did the first stem cell transplant in 1958 on 6 nuclear researchers who had been exposed to radiation. He was able to use bone marrow grafts to give these men extra stem cells, allowing their bodies to regenerate and heal from the exposure. He did it again in 1963, curing a patient of leukemia using bone marrow transplants.

Today, stem cell therapy is used to treat many health conditions. This exciting field of regenerative medicine can improve:

- Burns
- Heart Disease
- Cancer
- Osteoarthritis
- Stroke/brain damage
- Spinal cord injuries
- Type 1 Diabetes
- Alzheimer's Disease

- Parkinson's Disease
- Multiple Sclerosis (MS)
- Fibromyalgia
- Kidney Disease
- Corneal Regeneration in the eye

Some treatments involve using the patient's own bone marrow, encouraging the stem cells from the bone marrow to differentiate into a specific cell type, and inserting them back into the body where there is a problem.

Extracting stem cells from an embryo that is 3-5 days old produces about 150 pluripoint stem cells. Pluripoint means these stem cells can turn into any cell the body needs. These embryos are created through in-vitro fertilization in petri dishes and are not extracted from the mother's womb. In other countries such as Mexico, there are clinics that use voluntarily aborted embryos to get stem cells for patients who need them. Since this is a controversial topic in America, only embryos that are created in a lab are used for stem cell therapy.

There are also clinics that use amniotic fluid and tissue from the umbilical cord to obtain stem cells. These tissues are provided by willing mothers who have a live birth and choose to donate the placenta, umbilical cord, and amniotic sac to medicine instead of having them thrown away. These clinics are becoming increasingly popular in the US because of the ethical way these stem cells are derived along with how effective the treatments are.

Think about it this way, you are literally injecting yourself with young, almost brand-new cells that are healthy, vibrant, and able to turn into any specialized cell your body needs.

Treatments can be generalized through an IV drip that bathes the body in stem cells. They can also be specialized, injecting stem cells into a specific area that needs help with regeneration.

Essential Oils

Although essential oils aren't a cure-all for everything, they sure do have powerful effects on certain conditions.

For example, **Frankincense** and **Tea Tree Oil** have cured my skin cancer. I can confirm this from my own first-hand experience. I had a spot on my head that I could tell was becoming cancerous. I've had enough of my own skin cancers and have seen other people with skin cancer enough to know what it looks like, and I knew what this spot was.

I started treating it with Frankincense and Tea Tree oil (diluted in lotion) 3x per day. After a month, *the spot was* **GONE!**

Tea tree oil is also highly effective for treating acne, athlete's foot, and ringworms. It has antiseptic, antimicrobial, and anti-fungal properties as well.

Eucalyptus is another notorious healing plant, and not just in the alternative medicine world. One of the main active ingredients in Vicks VapoRub is eucalyptus. It is widely used for alleviating cold symptoms such as chest congestion while opening airways to improve breathing. Research shows that it does this by decreasing mucus in the body and expanding the bronchioles of the lungs.

An exciting 12-week study showed promising results of eucalyptus on asthma. Participants who were taking 600 mg of eucalyptol per day required 36% less medication to control their symptoms. If you have asthma, allergies, or any respiratory condition, consider diffusing this potent oil throughout your house. If you don't have a diffuser and need a quick solution to clear up congestion, boil water with eucalyptus oil in it and inhale the steam. Your breathing will get deeper, and your airways will open up, allowing for much needed symptom relief while struggling with sickness.

Peppermint oil is a powerful anti-inflammatory, anti-fungal, and antimicrobial which is why it is helpful for killing toe fungus. It also relieves headaches, improves digestion, and can reduce gut spasms.

Rosemary oil in addition to tasting absolutely delicious, improves brain function, increases hair growth, and reduces joint inflammation.

Essential oils have been used for many generations to improve health. Many of them kill viruses and bacteria while decreasing inflammation. Many of them greatly improve quality of life through the alleviation of anxiety and depression. Some of them will put a smile on your face right when you smell them, like **orange oil**.

I would greatly encourage you to do some research into essential oils and which ones could help your particular condition. Essential oils should be 100% pure therapeutic grade. Some can be taken internally, and others cannot. By incorporating these concentrated plant medicines into your health regimen, you will have a strong arsenal at your fingertips.

These are only a sampling of the amazing natural health solutions available to us. Many of these solutions are cheaper than traditional medical care and much more effective for certain conditions!

The truth of the matter is that doctors are not taught about all of these amazing health solutions. They are given a limited education in medical school that gives them the tools of surgery and pharmaceuticals. Remember, pharmaceutical companies provide funding for most medical schools, so it is not in their business interest to teach about treatments and cures from nature that they cannot patent!

So, when you go to your doctor and they either cannot find the problem or don't have an effective solution that treats the root cause of the problem, remind yourself that **THEY DON'T HAVE ALL THE ANSWERS.**

Think about it, even within the western medical system, we have specialists. There is so much to understand about the body and disease. One doctor cannot know everything about every condition. That's why physical therapists help people recover from musculoskeletal issues that primary doctors can only prescribe pain pills and muscle relaxants for.

Always ask questions and keep seeking solutions. Nature provides so many wonderful medicines for us if we are willing to seek them out and use them regularly. If your doctor cannot offer an effective solution, they probably just don't know about it. Doing your own research will open your eyes to the vast array of healing tools available. Connecting with an alternative medicine expert will give you access to a database of knowledge in the realm of natural treatment options. I have experimented with and seen incredible results from concentrated plant medicine such as chlorophyll, CBD, Niacin-amide, essential oils, and other whole food supplements.

Listen, don't think of me as some kind of hippie naturalist freak. Because I am definitely not! Pharmaceutical companies derive their medications FROM MOTHER NATURE! They then transform them into organic compounds for treatments. Some of these drugs are completely synthetic, meant to copy nature's creation, often with destructive side effects. Unfortunately, I am one of those people that tends to have significant side effects from medications. This has forced me to look for alternatives. So, who gets to benefit from my experimentations… YOU! Take it from me, I have found many that work *without* the annoying side effects.

However, don't forget, there's a time for pharmaceuticals as well.

Through a lifetime of seeking alternative healing solutions because of all my allergies and side effects to pharmaceuticals, I now believe that educating people on natural solutions is very beneficial for certain conditions and the combination of the two can be powerful and effective. Make sure to check with your pharmacist and your alternative medicine expert on the possible interactions of medications and remember, these are great options for a healthy lifestyle as well.

CHAPTER 13

THE TRUSTED HEALTH ADVOCATE

Imagine having someone to call when you're in a health crisis. Someone who knows the terminology and knows how to talk to doctors, other nurses, and insurance companies. Someone who can ask the right questions and get answers. Someone who can get to the bottom of what's going on in a very chaotic time. Someone to be the voice of reason and keep a calm, cool head during a very emotional time for you when maybe you can't think too clearly.

Get a Trusted Health Advocate

I have over a decade of experience in the emergency room as a nurse and have worked in several different units of the main hospital, along with surgical centers. I have dealt with a lot of intense and difficult medical situations.

Being a Firefighter/EMTII and an advanced diver-medic gave me a head start on knowing my stuff and being quick and effective. In the emergency room, I was no different. I would always fight for my patient's rights and call as many times as it took to reach the doctor. After losing a family member to medical negligence, I know how frustrating and heartbreaking it is to sit there and watch your loved one die because the staff is too busy (understaffed), careless, or jaded to save their life. It's the worst feeling in the world. I've suffered needlessly and seen my family members suffer at the hands of people who treat lives so nonchalantly.

My struggles have motivated me to use my knowledge and experience to help others navigate their health journeys through a jaded, overworked, and profit hungry medical system. It may sound harsh but it's the truth and the sooner you accept it, the sooner you will start taking responsibility for your own health.

It's obviously best to stay out of the hospital and doctor's office altogether, but should you find yourself in that unfortunate circumstance, get an advocate to fight for your rights and demystify your diagnosis. You very well may need someone to stand in your corner.

They can help you in the following ways:

- Actually listening to you and taking the time to understand what is going on with your health.

- Offer professional advice about which actions to take next - whether that be a diagnostic test, a treatment, and/or a lifestyle change.
- Come to the doctor with you if necessary as well as talk to him/her on the phone on your behalf.
- Record your office visits with consent and remind you to do the same if you are alone. They can also review these recordings through a professional lens.
- Demand the care you need if you are hitting walls with your healthcare providers.
- Fight for your rights while you are in the hospital.
- Make sure those who are caring for you are covered under your insurance.
- Keep an eye on your healthcare providers while you are receiving treatment to make sure they are doing all they can for you and not being negligent.
- Help you keep detailed documentation of your healthcare, diseases, medications, and treatments.
- Advocate for insurance coverage by getting on the phone with your insurance company.
- Help you decipher medical terminology and instructions.
- Make sure the staff is following infection prevention standards (cleansing hands on every entry). Nosocomial (hospital acquired) infection is common in the hospital environment.

- Be the strong, confident, demanding voice and presence you need when you are scared and emotional about your health.

Having a health advocate could literally mean the difference between life and death, as you have seen throughout this book. Many patients don't know what they don't know and as such cannot demand what they need. An advocate will know the technicalities of the system and what to watch out for. They also know what to ask for and how to be persistent enough to get you the care you need. They have learned how to talk to doctors to get them to act and know how to talk to fellow nurses to get the necessary information while holding them accountable for doing all they can for you.

The John Hopkins Medical website strongly suggests you come to all of your appointments with an advocate. Due to the complexities of our medical system, having someone by your side who can be calm, organized, knowledgeable, inquisitive, and assertive is now a necessity. Some are blessed with a family member in the medical field who can come with them to appointments. However, many are not lucky in this way, and this is the time to team up with someone who is knowledgeable about medicine to help you navigate your treatment plan.

Consider this statistic: In the United States, 27% of adults over age 60 live alone! Most of these people probably don't have anyone to go to their doctor's appointments with them. If you are one of those people, it is crucial that you have someone on your team to help you get the care you need. In addition, they can be your extra set of eyes and ears, helping you document what the doctors tell you and how they treat you. While many doctors are extremely caring people, there are some bad eggs in the system, and I want you to be protected from them.

No matter what your age, if you are experiencing negligence from the medical system and need help fighting for the care you deserve, an advocate will fight in your corner. Having someone experienced, knowledgeable, and professional on your team will give you a huge advantage in the care you receive. When doctors know someone is watching their every move, they tend to choose their actions more wisely.

Don't slip between the cracks of the medical system. Due to the high volume of patients, consistently short-staffed hospitals, and high rate of medical errors that occur in the US, keeping a health advocate on speed dial will give you a lifeline to grab onto when you need it. In a comprehensive study from 2016, researchers at John Hopkins found that an average of 250,000 people die needlessly as a result of medical errors each year.

My father was one of these people and the heartbreak it has caused my family is enormous. I don't want you to be another statistic. I want to get you the best care at the best time for the best outcome. And sometimes that means consistently fighting for your rights.

While the facts and statistics in this book are shocking and scary, it's important to understand the reality of the medical system in The United States. The more you know, the more you will realize the importance of educating yourself, asking questions, and having someone to ask for help who knows the system from the inside.

When dealing with a health problem or crisis, often your logical brain takes a back seat to your emotions. It is in these times when you need an advocate the most. You may be too weak physically or emotionally to fight for the care you need. You may even be unconscious in the emergency room and need someone to be your voice. No matter what stage of care you are in, with an advocate you have a better chance of getting the help you need for the best treatment possible.

This book exposes the state of our healthcare system, and I have risked my job to bring it to you. I am sure you have a story or two yourself. I can't stand to watch it anymore and not take action. Take the advice in this book and be happier and healthier because you did. It is my hope that all the information I provided in this book can get you started on a confident healthcare journey. Spread the word, it may save the life of someone you love and prevent the suffering of another.

BIOGRAPHY

Traci Konas is a registered nurse with 12 years of experience in the emergency department. After 2 years of working in the ER during COVID, she got burned out and started working in different units; GI lab, circulating in several types of ORs (operating rooms), PACU (recovery), Pre-op, IR (interventional radiology), and clinics. Before that, she was a Machinist, an Advanced Commercial Diver/Hyperbaric Paramedic, a Firefighter/EMTII, a Personal Trainer, and she has four college degrees: Associates of Oceaneering, Associates of Fire Science, Associates of Science, Associates of Nursing.

She graduated with honors (gold cords) for all her degrees. In commercial diving school she graduated top of the class, and in the fire academy she tied for top of the class. She somehow did all this while working full-time. She has won tournaments in women's boxing and competed and trained at the Olympic level.

She is also a pilot with the intention of leaving nursing to fly for the fire department. She is part of the Women in Aviation 99's Organization and has written and won a grant for a female wanting to learn to fly. She has always been an advocate and a fighter for her friends, family, and patients. She believes deeply in doing the right thing.

Traci Konas: RN - Your Trusted Health Advocate
Website: womendoing4women.com

SOURCES

Websites:

National Institutes of Health National Library of
     Medicine - nih.gov

Center for Disease Control and Prevention - cdc.gov

PubMed Central - ncbi.nlm.nih.gov

Mayo Clinic - mayoclinic.com

Medline Plus - medlineplus.gov

Department of Health and Human Services - hhs.gov

health.gov

WebMD.com

Healthline.com

ScienceDirect.com

BioMedCentral.com

MedicalNewsToday.com

statista.com

NPR Southern California

Open Secrets – opensecrets.org

JAMA Journal of the American Medical Association

NBC News - Gretchen Morgenson & Emmanuella Saliba

Book:

The Healing of America by T.R. Reid

<u>Contributors</u>

A SPECIAL THANK YOU TO

CO-WRITER: Tammy Bergstrom. While I was busy saving lives, Tammy helped me author this book.

<u>NURSES and DOCTORS</u>

Thank you to all the nurses and doctors that told me their stories to share with you!

Thank you to all the healthcare workers that try their best to be their patient's advocate. Your professionalism, compassion, and caring still mean something. KEEP AT IT!